Grandparents as Parents

Grandparents as Parents

A Survival Guide for Raising
a Second Family

SECOND EDITION

SYLVIE DE TOLEDO
DEBORAH EDLER BROWN

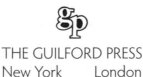

THE GUILFORD PRESS
New York   London

© 2013 Sylvie de Toledo and Deborah Edler Brown

Published by The Guilford Press
A Division of Guilford Publications, Inc.
72 Spring Street, New York, NY 10012
www.guilford.com

The following copyright holders have generously given permission to reprint from previously published works:

Senior Highlights for quotations from "Grandmothers Fill In for Drug-Abusing Parents" by Miriam Dobbin. Copyright 1990 by *Senior Highlights*. Used by permission.

Jessica Hernandez for her poem "Gracias to the Relatives of La Llorona," in *Grandparents as Parents: Filling the Gap*. Copyright 2012 by Jessica Hernandez. Used by permission.

Ethel Dunn for a quotation from "Those Wonderful Abuelas" in *Intergenerational Hookup*. Copyright 1993 by Ethel Dunn. Used by permission.

The information in this volume is not intended as a substitute for consultation with healthcare professionals. Each individual's health concerns should be evaluated by a qualified professional.

Printed in the United States of America

This book is printed on acid-free paper.

Last digit is print number: 9   8   7   6   5   4   3   2   1

Library of Congress Cataloging-in-Publication Data

De Toledo, Sylvie.
    Grandparents as parents: a survival guide for raising a
second family / Sylvie de Toledo and Deborah Edler Brown. —
Second edition.
        p.   cm.
    Includes bibliographical references and index.
    ISBN 978-1-4625-0919-5 (hardcover : alk. paper) —
ISBN 978-1-4625-0915-7 (pbk. : alk. paper)
    1. Grandparents as parents.   2.   Child rearing.
3. Intergenerational relations.   I. Brown, Deborah Edler.
II. Title.
    HQ759.9.D423 2013
    649'.1—dc23
                                                    2013003524

To the memory of Nikki de Toledo;
her son, Kevin;
and Andre and Ginette,
the grandparents who raised him

To grandparents everywhere
who are struggling to protect their grandchildren

We bereaved are not alone. We belong to the largest
company in all the world—the company of those
who have known suffering. When it seems that
our sorrow is too great to be borne, let us think of
the great family of the heavy-hearted into which
our grief has given us entrance, and, inevitably, we
will feel about us their arms, their sympathy, their
understanding.

—HELEN KELLER, *We Bereaved* (1929)

Contents

Section I
When the Second Shift Arrives

Section II
Through the Red Tape

Section III
Strength in Numbers

Appendices

Acknowledgments

No book of this scope can come to fruition without the support of a whole community—friends and family, grandparents, volunteers, and many outside experts who patiently offered insight and clarification—and we have been graced with help and heartfelt enthusiasm from some amazing individuals, both in the original book and in this second edition.

Our first thanks, now and always, must go to our families for their boundless support and encouragement. From the beginning of *Grandparents as Parents*, both the program and the book, Sylvie's family members have been case studies, cheerleaders, research assistants, volunteers, and benefactors. Her parents, Andre and Ginette de Toledo, set a world in motion when they opened their home to their suddenly orphaned grandson. Although Ginette is no longer with us, we feel their continuing presence in the organization and this book. The same is true for Sylvie's brother and sister-in-law, Philip and Alyce, and her nephew Kevin, who has been so open in sharing his story. We also owe an enormous debt of gratitude to Sylvie's husband, Jeffrey Hananel, and to their daughters, Ariella and Amelie. Their support, understanding, and patience allow Sylvie to continue her work with grandparents and relative caregivers in person and through these pages. It is equally hard to overstate the support of Deborah's family in this project. From the first draft, over 20 years ago, to this new edition, they have been a sounding board, an editorial board, and an ongoing pep rally. Her parents, Jack Brown and Ana Edler Brown, offered praise, advice, warm meals, and strong shoulders through the long process of writing the original book, and while Ana, too, is no longer with us, her encouragement and support persist in clear and subtle ways. We are still grateful to Deborah's brother Arthur, who carefully read and helped trim that first overgrown manuscript with insight and precision. Our families were, and remain, our bedrock. We could not have done any of this without them.

We owe much to our wonderful editor, Kitty Moore. In the first edition, she was our guide and our coach, whose enthusiasm and clear understanding focused our vision. Then she became our visionary, as her belief in the ongoing importance of this book led to the second edition you are holding now. We are so grateful to get to work with her twice.

JoBeth McDaniel was our matchmaker for this entire adventure. She introduced us to one another in 1991, and a happy meeting it was. If books have godmothers, JoBeth is ours.

We have been graced with guardian angels as well. We are indebted to attorneys Larry Hanna, Lara Holtzman, Pamela Mohr, Michael Salazar, Yolanda Vera, Peter Wright, Ted Youmans, and their assistants. They have all shared their time, knowledge, and resources to help us anchor this book in practical, accurate information about family law, government aid, and special education. All made time in their overcommitted schedules to read chapters and clarify subtle shifts of meaning. We are equally grateful to Phil Hopkins and Richard Sherer for jumping in as ad hoc editors, proofreaders, and consultants at several critical junctures; to Sheila Milnes for her insight on issues of childrearing; to Dr. Gigi Johnson for her expertise on technology and parenting; to Mary Weaver of Friends Outside for her compassionate insight regarding incarcerated parents; to Jill Rowland and Pamela Darr Wright for their help in unraveling the special education process; and to Eileen Pasztor and Joseph MacKenzie for helping us see the possibilities of peacemaking.

We also found angels and wise guides in such places as the Department of Health and Human Services, the Department of Agriculture, the Social Security Administration, the Child Welfare Information Gateway, the Census Bureau, and other government agencies. In particular, we must thank Julie Antoniou, Hans Billger, Dorothy Clark, Renee Ellis, Rose Kreider, Donna Lockhart, Sharon McKinley, Sandra McLeod, Gregg Porter,

Rich Proulx, Susan Ruiz, and Julie Yee. They fielded countless e-mails and phone calls to ensure that valuable information reaches the hands of families in need.

We also wish to thank Jacqueline Battle, Alice Bussiere, Jessica Cail, Leza Davis, Charles Ollinger, Anne Rutherford, Lori Waldinger, Dana Wilson, and Laurie Halderman for their time and insight. And special thanks go out to Josh Kroll of the North American Council on Adoptable Children for staying on the phone until a complex piece of legislation was distilled into three simple sentences.

No large project escapes last-minute panic, and two people in particular made themselves available up until the eleventh hour to answer late-night e-mails. Much thanks to Marjorie Shelvy of the Legal Aid Foundation of Los Angeles and Leslie Starr Heimov of the Children's Law Center of California. They were our lifelines.

Of course, none of this would have come together without the wonderful people at The Guilford Press. We thank them for their dedicated work, their enthusiasm, and their patience. They do the astonishing work of turning manuscripts into books—a combination of labor and magic that earns them our continuing gratitude.

We also want to thank Ethel Dunn, grandmother, colleague, and friend, who listened to fledgling chapters of the first edition by phone and who remains an advocate for grandparents and relative caregivers in every way that she can.

Thanks to Karen and Heidi Toffler, as well as Ken Stuckey from the Perkins School for the Blind, for doggedly tracking down the source of the marvelous quote from Helen Keller that starts the book; to Stuart Chapin, for offering up Carl Sandburg as a way to end it; and to Alvin Toffler for his lessons on how to put it all together.

Many others have helped out in quiet but important ways. Deborah would like to thank the close friends and extended family who have offered support, counsel, hugs, food, and incredible patience with the mental and physical absences of a writer in labor.

We are particularly grateful to the wonderful staff and board members of Grandparents As Parents (GAP), past and present, as well as to all the volunteers and interns who have helped GAP become the organization it is today. They have been our staunchest cheering section, and we couldn't have gotten this far without them. Special thanks go to Madelyn and Larry Gordon, who took GAP to a new level and, in doing so, broadened our readership, and to Barbara Wasson, who has been there almost from the start. We also need to thank Jessica Hernandez, who came on board to help with research and ended up adding her heart.

We deeply appreciate the efforts of all the journalists, bloggers, and talk-show hosts who are shedding light on grandparent issues and of all the advocates who are working to improve the plight of grandparents and relative caregivers, as well as of children in general.

Finally, no thanks would be complete without acknowledging the countless grandparents and relative caregivers who have so generously shared their stories with us. It was their faces, and the faces of the children they are raising, that kept us going. They were our heartbeat and our light.

Preface

It's hard to believe that it has been 18 years since *Grandparents as Parents* was first published. So much has changed in that time. So many things have happened that I could never have imagined when Deborah and I began writing the first edition more than two decades ago.

Personally, I met and married an amazing man, Dr. Jeffrey Hananel, who realized that if he married me, he was getting a world of grandparents in the bargain, and he said yes to all of us. I became the mother of two astonishing daughters, Ariella and Amelie, who are growing up as part of one of the world's largest and most eclectic families. We've also helped raise a couple of kids from the Grandparents As Parents (GAP) community. And I lost my mother who, with my father, set me on this journey when they took in my nephew Kevin so many years ago.

GAP, the organization, has also changed dramatically in the last 18 years. What began as a few grandparents in my living room—and had reached nine groups by 1995—has grown into a professional nonprofit with offices, a CEO, a staff, and generous donors. Twenty groups, including three Spanish-speaking ones, now serve families in Los Angeles County, and they are composed of much more than grandparents. We also have a teen group and a group for grandparents who are raising teenagers. As more and more children need safe homes, we have reached out to help the aunts, uncles, great-grandparents, cousins, and adult siblings who have joined the ranks of relative caregivers. And while GAP still provides emotional and practical support, we have shifted from political activism to education and advocacy, with a curriculum to help educate relative caregivers and our own caregiver center at the Edelman Children's Court. What this means is that, as the organization begins its 25th year, we spend less time protesting on the courthouse steps and more time inside, where attorneys, judges, and social workers recognize us as a resource for families.

Sadly, there are more of those families than ever before. Changes in the world at large have only served to increase the number of grandparents raising grandchildren. The crises that create grandfamilies—drug and alcohol abuse, incarceration, violence, disease, and suicide—continue to undermine parent–child relationships, and many have gotten worse. Crack was the big epidemic when we first wrote this book; now it's meth and pharmaceuticals. Who knows what it will be in the years to come? And while the drugs keep changing, the problems do not; the number of drug-exposed infants has more than doubled since the mid-1990s,[1] as have child deaths due to child abuse and neglect,[2] and the number of incarcerated mothers.[3] There are also new problems that challenge families. In a post-9/11 world, war and military deployment have increased the demands on relatives, as has the stress and joblessness brought on by recession.

Meanwhile, grandparents are raising grandkids in a world that looks radically different from the one in which they raised their own children. Many of today's grandparents were still young parents when this book first came out. There was no Internet, no smartphones, no texting, no Facebook, no Pinterest. Social networking was still something you did at a cocktail party, and child safety meant not talking to strangers on the street.

What has not changed, however, are the feelings and dilemmas grandparents experience when they suddenly become parents again. I can pick up any article on grandparents raising grandchildren, from any time in the last 25 years, and the stories are the same. They could be speaking in yesterday's meeting.

All of this was on our minds as we approached this second edition. The book you hold in your hands has been updated to reflect current data, laws, procedures, and technology, but it retains all the stories and suggestions that made it a support group in a book. One chapter has been cut.

The first edition featured a mini-manual on political action, which is not included here. The Internet has dramatically altered that arena, and other people are carrying that torch better than we can.

On the other hand, we have added practical new advice throughout the book, including a section on raising children in a high-tech world and an expanded section on dealing with incarcerated parents. For those of you who are starting or running support groups, we have added a look at GAP 2.0 and, just for its unexpected beauty, a poem written by a young social work intern, inspired by the relative caregivers in the groups she helped facilitate.

Readers of the first edition might also find a slight change in tone in some chapters. From the late 1980s to the mid-1990s, grandfamilies were still a new social phenomenon, and their issues represented unfamiliar terrain for social workers, attorneys, and judges, who were used to dealing with unrelated foster parents. As a result, relative caregivers often found themselves treated with suspicion and resistance. They felt like they were waging a war ... to protect their grandchildren and to be seen and heard. It was a dynamic time. Grandparent groups formed national and local coalitions, rallied on capitol steps, and met with legislators to educate people about themselves and their issues. Some people called it "Granny's March on Washington," and most of the advances that have helped grandparents came out of those efforts. But it was hard work, and some of our language reflected that feeling of being under siege.

While individual grandparents may still feel that way—understandably so—and while many support groups are still deeply engaged in educating and advocating for grandparent concerns, the good news is that things are slowly changing. Google "grandparents raising grandchildren" today, and you get a plethora of hits, from meeting notices, blogs, and news items to master's theses and studies in professional journals. "Kinship care" has become a commonly used term, and in many areas, efforts are being made to make the legal system more accessible to relatives. More importantly, society has begun to acknowledge the existence of grandparent families and the importance of extended family in a child's life, as both a heart bond and a safety net.

Grandparents and relative caregivers are finally being counted, literally, by the U.S. Census. That creates the kinds of statistics that help drive awareness, services, and policy change. The Adoption and Safe Families

Act of 1997 marked a fundamental change in the way we think about child welfare, foster care, and adoption. It shifted the focus away from a policy of reuniting children with parents as the first goal of dependency and replaced it with an emphasis on children's health and safety. Eleven years later, another act would expand that focus on a child's well-being and bring extended family clearly into the discussion. The Fostering Connections to Success and Increasing Adoptions Act of 2008 includes a list of provisions to improve the lives of children and youth in foster care. It also shines a light on the importance of family by requiring that states look for and notify relatives when a child is removed, promoting permanent families through relative guardianship and adoption, and allocating funds to create nationwide "kinship navigator programs" to help relative caregivers access legal, financial, and government assistance, as well as support groups and other critical services. As I said, a lot of changes in two decades.

Eighteen years ago, Deborah and I held the first edition of *Grandparents as Parents* in our hands. The books were like new babies; we didn't expect them to smell so good! Readers would approach us at conferences and ask, "How do you know what goes on in my house?" Social workers and attorneys snapped it up to get some insight into this "new" population. And now you are holding Edition Two. It is my wish that it continue to do its work—reaching grandparents and professionals who worry about children in need, creating understanding and collaboration, and functioning as an A–Z handbook to help you on your journey of loving and protecting the children in your care.

SYLVIE DE TOLEDO
June 1, 2012

Grandparents as Parents

Introduction

I n 1983 my sister committed suicide. She locked the doors of her house and overdosed on pills that had been prescribed for depression. She didn't leave a note. She did leave an eight-year-old son. She was 27 years old.

I was away in graduate school, finishing a master's degree in social work. My sister and I had a standing phone date. Every Saturday morning at six o'clock I would call her. My nephew would be asleep, and we could talk without interruption. As a single mother, my sister didn't have much time without interruption. Since Kevin would wake up at some point during the call, I would talk with him, too. Nikki and I were close in age—one year and one week apart—and we were best friends.

That Saturday I called and called, but there was no answer. I finally called my parents to see if they knew where Nikki was. Kevin had spent the previous night at my brother's house and was scheduled to stay with my parents that night to give his mother a free weekend. But she hadn't said anything about going out. We decided they should use the spare key and go in. It didn't work. One lock wouldn't open. It was the one Nikki locked from inside. "She's in there, Mom," I said. "I know she's in there." My parents had the police knock down the door. Nikki was there, but it was too late. I caught the next plane to Los Angeles (by this time, it was early the next morning).

Overnight, we went from a family of five adults to one of four, a hand

1

with a missing finger. We were devastated, and we were in shock. Grief had joined our family.

And then there was Kevin.

Kevin had always been the family child. Nikki dropped out of school at 18 to have him. His father was never part of the picture.

And although Nikki and Kevin had their own apartment, my parents, my brother, and I were always helping out in different ways. Kevin was lovable and he was difficult. Now, at the age of eight, he was parentless.

There was no question of what to do. My parents took Kevin in, and in that moment they became part of a family much larger than ours, although we didn't know it then. They joined the growing ranks of grandparents who are raising their grandchildren.

The media call them "silent saviors,"[1] "recycled parents,"[2] and, when they are also caring for aging parents, "the sandwich generation."[3] At a time in their lives when they expected to be traveling, enjoying hobbies, and doing everything they had put on hold while raising their first set of children, they find themselves back in a routine of bottles, diapers, and PTA meetings, sometimes 30 years after they last had kids in the house. Instead of doting grandparents who can spoil and coddle and send the kids back to Mom and Dad, they are surrogate parents with all the responsibilities of raising another set of children.

Some are as young as 35, others are in their 80s. Some are even great-grandparents and stepgrandparents. They cross economic lines, social lines, and religious lines. They become caregivers because of abandonment, neglect, and abuse, as well as death by illness, accident, suicide, and murder. In some instances their adult children are in jail or mentally ill. In other instances a single parent is unemployed or deployed by the military. But the most common reason grandparents raise grandchildren, by far, is parental drug and alcohol abuse.

The kids these grandparents get are troubled, burdened with everything from emotional, behavioral, psychological, medical, and academic problems to physical disabilities from a parent's prenatal drug and alcohol abuse.

Almost six million children live in the homes of their grandparents. Even so, too many grandparents think they are in this alone. Not a day goes by that I don't get calls, letters, and e-mails from grandparents around the country who are looking for a group, a piece of information, or someone to listen to them who will understand their concerns. The letters come typed, written, and scribbled in crayon, on everything from napkins to torn scraps of paper. Some write "Dear Ms. de Toledo" or "Dear GAP [Grandparents As Parents]" and tell their stories; others just write "Help!" One grandparent in Georgia seemed to say it for all of them when he wrote, "I took my grandson when his mother died six years ago. Ten months ago, his dad died. We need people. My friends call once in a while but don't come around. We are like in a world alone. We need people."

This book had to be written because there was absolutely nothing out there back then to answer those letters. I talked to thousands of grandparents across the country and realized there was nothing to help these families. People asked me about resources, and because I had nowhere to refer them, I would offer to help start a group in their community.

Before I started my first Grandparents As Parents support group in 1987, I searched a number of libraries for information on grandparents raising grandchildren. I was looking for a foundation. If there was material out there, I didn't want to reinvent the wheel. Unfortunately, I didn't find anything in the professional literature, let alone the consumer press.

By the time the first edition came out, GAP had grown into an organization of nine support groups across southern California and had already helped start hundreds of others throughout the country. Local grandparent groups across the United States had joined forces to create a strong national voice on grandparent issues. Researchers had begun to study the grandparenting phenomenon, and a few authors had published books on the changing role of grandparents.[4] Still, there was nothing out there that addressed the broad spectrum of grandparent issues in one place.

And for all the websites and manuals that have cropped up in the intervening years, there are still few places that hold a grandparent's hand so well, through so many of the twists and turns of second-time parenting.

So, this is *GAP: The Book.* It is part map, part dictionary, and something of a group hug—a handbook for all grandparents who are raising grandchildren, to help them through the stressful times. Inside you will find descriptions of many of the common problems grandparents face when they take in their grandchildren, as well as practical suggestions for how to cope. You will also find basic information on topics such as government aid, court proceedings, and special education. I hope this book will help get you through the alphabet soup of AAP, SSI, IEP, ISFP, WIC, and CPS. In these pages you will find guidelines for finding and forming groups, two sure ways of empowering yourself in a situation that can often make you feel powerless. Here, as in a GAP meeting, I offer support, resource information, and a professional perspective. But it is the other grandparents who will let you know you are not alone, that you can get through this, that whatever you are going through is normal. In the following pages, you will hear their voices and their stories.*

Second-time parenting can be pretty grim sometimes. You face troubled children, uncooperative parents, and a bureaucracy that may not understand your new role or support your new needs. This book does not shy away from those stark realities. It does not suggest that if you follow a prescribed set of steps, your problems will vanish. Life isn't that simple. It does, however, offer hope. By raising grandchildren, you offer them a new future. By learning your options you give yourself choices. By recognizing problems you learn when to adapt and when to fight back. And by joining forces you create hope for the grandparents who follow you.

A NOTE TO PROFESSIONALS WHO WORK WITH GRANDPARENTS

I hope this book will also provide insight for people who work with grandparents: mental health professionals, teachers, doctors, attorneys—anyone who comes in contact with grandparents raising grandchildren and children being raised by their grandparents.

I receive frequent requests from educators and mental health professionals about how to develop groups for grandparents. My work is based on years of observing and doing therapeutic work with grandparent families, as well as on personal experience with my own family. This treatment incorporates many aspects: crisis intervention, individual needs assessment, meeting survival needs of individual families, modeling cop-

---

*So as to avoid using sexist language—and so as not to encumber the book with an excessive use of "he or she" and "him or her"—we have decided to alternate between masculine and feminine pronouns. We have attempted to do this consistently, and have tried to avoid ascribing the male and female pronouns in a stereotypical way.

ing skills, teaching problem-solving techniques, and supportive therapy. Some of the work I do is nontraditional for mental health professionals, but I believe it is critical for grandparent families.

Chapter 14 specifically addresses support groups for grandparents: how to find them, how to start them, and what programs and principles have been successful for GAP. The chapter is designed to assist both grandparents and mental health professionals in the rewarding process of developing groups; I hope it helps you.

HOW TO READ THIS BOOK

Grandparents as Parents is designed as both a book and a manual. You can read it front to back, following the grandparent stories that span the chapters, or you can turn to whatever chapter addresses your immediate questions, without worrying about order.

The book is divided into three sections. Section I, "When the Second Shift Arrives," covers the personal and social aspects of raising grandchildren: the changes, the feelings, and the problems of adult children, grandchildren, and family in general. It starts with an overview of the recent rise in grandparents as parents and looks at some of the myths about the phenomenon. Section II, "Through the Red Tape," addresses the bureaucratic part of raising grandchildren, the legal issues, and the availability of government assistance and special education. And Section III, "Strength in Numbers," focuses on the larger community of grandparents as parents and provides information on finding, starting, and nurturing support groups.

Grandparents as Parents represents the work of two authors—myself and journalist Deborah Edler Brown—yet it is written from one point of view. The reason is simple: We wanted this to be a comfortable, personal book, and years of working with grandparents has given me an intimate understanding of the subject. As you read through the following chapters, the voice and perspective you encounter will be mine. I hope they help you.

When my sister ended her life, a whole world ended for me. And another one opened. Somehow, when I see the growth of GAP, I feel that something positive is coming from the death of my sister. There is a special place in my heart for grandparents who are parenting again. You all deserve a gold medal for what you're doing. You have sacrificed to be here, and my heart goes out to you.

Sylvie de Toledo

Grandparents as Parents accurately conveys the themes that are the most central to grandparents who are raising grandchildren, but the names and identifying characteristics of most of the grandparents and grandchildren mentioned in the book have been changed in order to protect their privacy.

SECTION I

When the Second Shift Arrives

1

Unplanned Parenthood

"WHY ME?"

Becoming a parent again is not a first choice. It's a last alternative.
—*Barbara Kirkland, founder of
Grandparents Raising Grandchildren*[1]

Sometimes the call comes at night, sometimes on a bright morning. It may be your child, the police, or child protective services. "Mama, I've messed up. . . . " "We're sorry. There has been an accident. . . . " "Mrs. Smith, we have your grandchild. Can you take him?" Sometimes you make the call yourself—reporting your own child to the authorities in a desperate attempt to protect your grandchild from abuse or neglect. Often the change is gradual. At first your grandchild is with you for a day, then four days, a month, and then two months as the parents slowly lose control of their lives. You start out baby-sitting. You think the arrangement is temporary. You put off buying a crib or moving to a bigger apartment. Then you get a collect call from jail—or no call at all.

But whether the arrival is slow or sudden, at some point it dawns on you: You are no longer watching your grandchildren, you are raising them. Take the *grand* out of *grandparent;* you are parenting again, and your life will never be the same.

Emily Petersen knew her pregnant daughter-in-law, Sheila, was a drug addict. She knew the young woman was using drugs throughout her entire pregnancy, and she was prepared to see the effects in her newborn granddaughter—the stiff body, the frantic eyes, the shakes. What Emily was not prepared for was becoming a mother again at 59. But when she and her husband, Carter, arrived at the hospital to see the baby, they found a social worker and two bodyguards outside the hospital room. Sheila had been arrested on drug charges, and the baby was being removed. The social worker asked Emily if she would be willing to take the child. "I came in to visit a baby," Emily told her. "I didn't come to take a baby home." But her son was in tears, begging them not to send Amanda into foster care, and neither Emily nor Carter could stand the idea of not knowing where their granddaughter was. A week later they filed for custody.

Ivy Johnson had not seen her daughter Rachel in four years; she had never even met her youngest granddaughter. They lived in Arizona and had no money to travel. Then Rachel left her husband and came home with her kids. The minute she came to the door, Ivy knew something more was wrong. Within three days Rachel was diagnosed with liver cancer. Seven months later she died, leaving Ivy to raise five young grandchildren in a one-bedroom apartment.

There is nothing new about a grandparent raising a child in a crisis. For centuries grandparents have taken over when their grandchildren were orphaned by disease or war or when financial troubles split a family. They have also stepped in to support single mothers and widowed or divorced parents of both sexes. Moreover, there is a proud tradition of intergenerational families in working-class neighborhoods as well as in African American and Hispanic communities of all income levels.[2]

What *is* new are the numbers: of grandparents, of grandchildren, of crises. According to the U.S. Census Bureau, approximately 7.8 million children under 18 (one in 10) were living with at least one grandparent in 2009—a 64 percent increase in almost two decades.[3] About half of those children—about 5.4 million—lived in the grandparent's home, and nearly two million had no parents present at all.[4] And the real numbers are probably higher: Many grandparents don't acknowledge or recognize that they are taking full-time care of their grandchildren; perhaps they only watch them four days a week or are ashamed to admit that their own children can't parent. Many don't believe the situation is permanent. "What's wrong with my generation that we can't or won't raise our kids?"

asks one young mother in Texas. The answer paints a picture of growing tragedy in American families.

AMERICA'S CHILDREN IN CRISIS

Grandparents raise grandchildren for one reason: because the children need someone to raise them. It was true a hundred years ago, and it is true today. Most grandparents had other plans for this stage of their lives; raising another child wasn't part of them. To quote a grandmother in Oregon: "The bottom line of this whole thing is I didn't need another child; the child needed a mother."

On the other hand, there are many reasons why these children need their grandparents. One writer pinned the cause on what he called the four D's: drugs, divorce, desertion, and the death of a parent.[5] Indeed, illness, accident, suicide, and murder leave numerous children without parents to care for them, and drugs and alcohol shatter thousands of young families each year. But child abuse, incarceration, and teen pregnancy also contribute to the growing number of children without stable homes, while joblessness, economic insecurity, and military deployment of a single parent or both parents can create even more need for grandparental support. Most families suffer from a combination of problems, and the rate at which all these problems are growing is frightening. The statistics point to a nation of children in crisis:

- One in two marriages ends in divorce. More than one million children experience divorce each year.[6] Some parents go on to remarry with little interest in their own offspring.
- Teen pregnancy rates are high.[7] Nearly half a million children are born to teenagers in the United States each year.[8]
- Over three million reports of child abuse are made in the United States each year, but each report can involve multiple children.[9]
- The prison population has exploded. Over 50 percent of inmates— men and women—are parents of dependent children.[10]
- More women are abusing drugs. Every year between 550,000 and 750,000 children are born with drugs in their systems.[11]
- Between 7,000 and 12,000 children a year lose a parent to suicide.[12]

Many of these children end up in foster care, separated from their siblings and cared for by strangers. But the foster care system itself is in crisis, with a rising demand for care and a shrinking number of qualified foster parents.

All this leaves grandparents, and other relatives, as one of the few safety nets protecting these children from an increasingly precarious future. In fact, as of 2011, over 50 percent of children placed in out-of-home care in Los Angeles County were placed with grandparents and other relative caregivers.[13]

Whether your grandchild lives with you because of drugs, death, military deployment, abuse, or abandonment, there are certain factors that are *not* responsible for this second parenthood, despite what people think.

THE MYTHS

There are several reactions that appear, like clockwork, each time a discussion turns to grandparents as parents. They are assumptions that allow people to explain away the phenomenon, to pretend that it doesn't touch them, and to put the blame, somehow, on the victim:

"It's a black problem, right?"

"It's a poor problem—or an urban problem—isn't it?"

"Well, those grandparents probably deserve it if they messed up their first set of kids."

These biases exist as much in the judge deciding a custody case as in the person watching the news. They are responsible for much of the intolerance you may encounter as you try to find help for yourself and protection for your grandkids. These assumptions imply that the "second-time parenting" is something that happens to someone else, when the sad truth is that each and every grandparent is only one or two tragedies away from the decision to raise a grandchild.

If you and the children you care for are ever to receive the help you desperately need and deserve, we must see through these myths and acknowledge the true breadth and scope of the grandparenting phenomenon.

Myth 1: It's an Urban, Minority Problem

Say "grandparents as parents" to people, and, for many, certain pictures come to mind: Black faces. Brown faces. City dwellers. Families in poverty. These pictures are not inaccurate, but they are incomplete. Raising grandchildren is not strictly an urban, poor, or minority problem. If it were, it would be no less of a social crisis. But it is not. It is an international phenomenon. Grandparents are raising grandchildren in places as different from one another as New York City, Honolulu, London, and Paducah, Kentucky. In recent years, I have met professionals working with relative caregivers in Canada, Puerto Rico, and The Netherlands, and I've heard stories from such far-flung places as Australia and Tanzania. I doubt there is a country in the world where you would *not* find grandparents raising grandchildren.

Parenting a grandchild is a necessity born of tragedy, and tragedy has no regard for location, ethnicity, religion, class, or race. Grandparenting is color-blind. It is also class-blind. The same can be said of the drug epidemic that drives it.

Drugs and alcohol account for more than 80 percent of grandparent families. They show up combined with teen pregnancy, abuse, neglect, and abandonment. They show up in connection with incarceration and murder. Moreover, suburban, middle-class, and white families are not immune from addiction; they only hide it better. Middle-class addicts may have better access to private drug treatment programs and may be less likely to end up in jail. Private doctors may be less likely to question pregnant women about drugs and alcohol than are inner-city doctors in public clinics and county hospitals. To quote one grandmother, "Drugs affect us all, whether you live in the streets or in a mansion." So does tragedy. Both are indiscriminate. Who you are and where you live are not to blame for your situation, and neither are you.

Myth 2: It's Your Fault

Grandparents hear it all the time. "If you raised a drug addict, how can we trust you to raise this child?" It's a question that hangs in the air, spoken or unspoken. It floats through the legal system, where judges and social workers may wonder to what extent the grandparents are responsible for the adult child's inability to parent.

It even haunts grandparents themselves: "What did we do wrong?" "Is this our fault?" "Are we grandparenting because we failed as parents?" One grandmother feels guilty because she worked nights as a nurse; she fears that may be why her daughter is on drugs. Another is afraid that she didn't love her son enough, that perhaps she wasn't there when he needed her, and that it drove him to drugs.

Let me set the record straight. You did not raise your children to be drug addicts, welfare mothers, prostitutes, or even irresponsible parents. Did you make mistakes in childrearing? Probably. Most people do. Are there things you could have done differently? Certainly. We all have 20/20 hindsight. But you did not cause your child's addiction or the abuse or neglect of his or her own child. You did the best you could with what you knew at the time. Again and again, I see families where two or three children grow up to be upstanding citizens and competent parents and one loses control of her life: The New Jersey grandparents who raised a talented musician, a successful accountant, and a young woman who became addicted to drugs. The Montana grandparents who raised three boys—an architect, a county sheriff, and a drug addict. How are these grandparents to be blamed for their children's failings?

Even when child abuse or addiction seems to run in a family—and these problems can be cyclical—grown people have a choice about whether to continue the cycle or break it. There are many adults who were abused as children who do not grow up to be abusers and many children of addicts who take a different path. "It is the use of substance that creates substance abuse problems," says one psychologist. "We have a whole society that has problems with that, and that is certainly not the making of any particular grandparent."[14]

No one makes a person take drugs, abandon a baby, or abuse a child. Whatever choices you made as parents are past you. You did the best you could with the tools you had. Your children are now adults, and they are making their own choices.

THE REASONS FOR GRANDPARENTING

There are many complicated reasons why grandchildren need grandparents to care for them. But, in the end, the reasons you take them in are straightforward and simple: love, duty, and the bonds of family. Over and over I hear the same refrains: "We want to keep the kids together." "We're all he has." Often you are the only one standing between your grandchild and foster care. I have seen many grandparents disrupt their lives, their finances, and their health to keep their grandchildren together and away from care by strangers.

Anne Sutter's grandson Gregory was born in a crack house, and his mother was arrested on drug-related charges. At 60 years of age and on a limited income, Anne was not prepared to care for an infant, but there was that tiny baby, born stiff and distorted, with drugs in his system, and Anne couldn't say no. She recalls, "I looked at him and thought to myself, 'Nobody else will love my baby; they will look at him and think he's a thing.'"

"I'd do it all again," says another grandmother, even though her boyfriend left her when the grandkids arrived. "You do it because you're family. Nowhere, no way can you ever replace that."

A grandfather calls it a labor of love: "I don't think I could live with it if they went to somebody else."

2

Taking Immediate Action

I live with my grandma because my mom left me on a hotel
bench to go get a cup of coffee. You're not supposed to leave
babies by theirselves.

—*Erica, age seven*

Late one Saturday night the phone call came: Leah Croft's 18-month-old grandson had been left unattended in an apartment. The little boy had tried to feed himself dry oatmeal and had started choking. Someone had called the police, and child protective services had removed the baby from his mother. They wanted Leah to take him in. Leah was already raising her daughter Jill's six-year-old twins but, because of Jill's transient lifestyle, had only seen her grandson three times before that night. At 10:30 P.M., Josh arrived in the arms of a social worker. Dressed in a sleeper that had the legs cut off because it was too small for him, he had no socks, no shoes, no bottle, no car seat, and only the diaper he was wearing. The next day was a frenzy. In addition to buying baby supplies, Leah had to find a sitter so she could go to work Monday morning. She had to buy diapers with her credit card because she didn't have enough cash. No one from social services told her she was eligible for government aid for the baby, and when she called to ask about it, she got the runaround. "For five months I didn't get one dime," she fumes. "Not one dime!"

Whether a grandchild arrives in one night or over a period of months, few grandparents plan, anticipate, or prepare for a second parenthood. Your home and lifestyle are geared to adult living. You are not expecting these children or these changes. Instead of one small baby, you may, like Ivy Johnson, acquire several children at once, all at different ages with different needs. You may find yourself facing complex emotional, financial, and legal situations that you are rarely prepared for. You may have to resolve problems overnight that most parents address over a period of months, if not years. While each family has different needs, there are a few things that every grandparent should look into as soon as possible:

• *Consider other options.* Some grandparents don't have the health or resources to raise a second family, but they do it anyway. A few, however, have been able to place their grandchild with another family member, perhaps a son or daughter who already had children and was willing to raise this child as well. If you have family members who can help out, you might consider letting them step in or at least sharing the responsibility with them. Parenting your grandchildren not only disrupts your life but deprives the children of grandparents who can spoil them and send them home for their parents to deal with. The children have already lost an important relationship with their parents; now they are losing a precious relationship with you.

Most grandparents, however, don't have other options, and the majority don't want to burden their other adult children. Their only choice is to gear up for the changes and the feelings that come along with raising grandchildren.

• *Keep records.* One of the most important things you can do when your grandchildren arrive is to start taking notes. I know that buying notebooks and pens sounds more like preparation for school than for grandparenting, but when you take in your grandchildren, you become more than a surrogate parent; you become their advocate. You may be the only voice speaking solely for their safety and their interests, trying to protect their rights in court, in school, and in the welfare system. You are the one who knows that Dad has a drug problem and that the children are being neglected and/or abused whenever they are with him. You are the one who knows that Max throws tantrums in school after Mom comes to visit. Unfortunately, few people will want to listen to the grandparent, which is why you must document everything. The more organized you are, the better your chances that those who listen will believe you (see the section on documentation in Chapter 5).

You will also want to use your notebooks to set yourself up as a kind of central headquarters. Throughout this book you will find lists of the kinds of records you will need to keep: names and phone numbers of attorneys, social workers, and welfare workers connected to your grandchild; the names of their supervisors; and information for school, for doctors, and for the welfare office. The more organized you are from the start, the less crazy you may feel later on.

Remember, the best advocate is an organized one. If you ever need to lock horns with the system, you want to be ready. Keep records of the professionals you talk to and what they tell you. Create a paper trail of letters and documents. Keep dates and times of conversations. Try to write letters when you can and keep copies. Knowledge is power; it may be the only power you have. But nothing you know will do any good if you can't present it in a clear, convincing fashion.

• *Sort out the legal maze.* Your grandchildren are family, pure and simple. However, family is also a legal relationship, with rights and responsibilities that can be determined by the courts. Your rights toward your grandchildren will mostly depend on why they are with you. As soon as possible, find out what your legal rights are in this situation and how you can best protect them. Chapter 10 offers a broad overview of custody issues to get you started, but you will probably want to consult an attorney or other legal professional about your individual case.

• *Look into financial aid.* Raising children is expensive. Raising children on a fixed retirement income is expensive and stressful. And raising children on a fixed welfare income, as some grandparents must do, can make you crazy. Whatever obligations you feel you have toward your grandchildren, and I know there are many, you do not have an obligation to support them financially. Financial support is a parent's responsibility. If parents don't fulfill that responsibility, their children are entitled to government assistance.

Many grandparents are reluctant to look to the government for help or don't believe they qualify. They have never asked for help before, and the process mystifies them. Still, while government benefits won't make you rich, every little bit helps, especially Medicaid. As soon as you can, find out what assistance is available to your grandchildren. (For more on government aid, see Chapter 12.)

• *Get financial advice.* Even with government assistance, second-time parenting will shake up your financial world, impacting everything from immediate cash flow to retirement plans. Some grandparents have to reallocate funds, work longer, or return to work in order to provide for their grandkids. If you can, consider meeting with a financial planner or counselor to help you evaluate your immediate and long-term needs. It doesn't matter how much, or how little, you have; professional guidance could help you better navigate the new financial waters ahead.

• *Arrange for medical care.* One of the biggest expenses with children is health care. Immunizations and the treatment of colds, earaches, and childhood sprains can add up to a small fortune. Many grandparents are shocked to discover that their insurance companies will not add grandchildren to their policies. However, the children can often be covered by Medicaid. Again, apply early (see Chapter 12).

• *Keep medical records.* Accurate medical records can be critical when you raise a child. Few children arrive at grandma's house with records of any kind, but if you can somehow acquire them, they will make your life easier. For instance, have your grandchildren had all their immunization shots? If you don't know, you'll have to start all over. Many grandchildren have had to be reimmunized because of lost records. If the children come to you from a foster care placement or group home, ask the social worker for their medical records. At the very least, try to compile a family medical history based on what you do know about your family. You never know what information could be important later on.

• *Enroll them in school.* If you can keep your grandchild in the same school or day care facility, consider yourself lucky. It's one less change for the child and less stress for you. If not, try to get school records and reports of any special education programs transferred with the child (see Chapter 13). Special education plans should be transferable to the new school, even if it is in another state. Granted, school is much easier to handle in an intact family that was hit by crisis, like a death, than in a family where the parents were on drugs and the child rarely made it to school. Just do the best you can.

• *Consider counseling.* Few children are raised by their grandparents for happy reasons. Many grandchildren arrive with emotional, psychological, behavioral, or academic difficulties and/or with physical problems caused by parental abuse or prenatal drug exposure. Most arrive suffering from grief, loss, and abandonment. If your grandchildren are old enough to talk about feelings and events, consider getting them into counseling. Even if they are too young for counseling on their own, you can work with a counselor on their behalf, learning techniques to help them cope with the situation. I have worked with a number of grandparents to address a child's temper tantrums or inability to sleep in his own bed. These children have all had their lives somehow shattered. A support group or family counseling can start the process of gluing them back together.

• *Find your own emotional support.* Raising a second family is stressful and exhausting. It wears on your time, your energy, your finances, and your spirit. Like your grandchildren, you have suffered loss. But you also shoulder the responsibilities. Don't try to do this alone. Look around at your resources. Who can be your emotional support? Whom can you turn to for help? My parents were fortunate. They never worried about baby-sitters because my brother and I were there, although they did worry about burdening us. Many families really are alone. Perhaps your new circumstances involve your only child, or your other children live far away or don't support your taking in the grandchildren. If that is true, you may have to look elsewhere for support. Try other grandparents, a support group, or even a therapist to blow off steam, but do look for help.

• *Join a group.* You are not alone. Everything you are feeling is completely normal. And help is available. I can't stress enough how important it is for you to understand this. There are other families just like yours, waiting to put their arms around you and help you through the transitions to this new reality. They've been where you are. They know how you feel. And they can save you time and frustration as you navigate the legal and emotional maze of second parenthood. I've seen grandparents accompany fellow grandparents to court, help out with practical things like clothes and food, even temporarily take kids in when Grandma got sick. Take care of yourself—and, by extension, your grandchild—by joining a support group as soon as possible. You don't have to do this alone. (For more on finding and forming support groups, see Chapter 14.)

3

Your Lifestyle

CHANGED AND CHALLENGED

> It is not the American Dream of a grandparent to raise a
> second family.
>
> —*Letter from Texas*

Beth Grafton's life was sweet. Her six children were grown, and she was in a wonderful marriage to Alan, the man of her dreams. Alan had his own business and a comfortable amount of savings. Beth managed a clothing store. If they needed something, they bought it. Alan's father, whom they had nursed for two years, had died the year before, leaving them with the house to themselves and time to rekindle their marriage. After years of renting they were getting ready to buy a home. On weekends Alan would shop and play golf; Beth would do yard work, work on crafts, and visit their grandchildren. In the evenings they would go out to dinner or dancing. Every other month they would join a group of friends on Cape Cod for the weekend.

And they had future plans. They dreamed of taking cruises, since neither one had ever been on one, and of traveling through the United States together. They worried about their adult children but knew they couldn't control their children's lives.

Then the unthinkable happened: Their daughter Ellen was stabbed to death by an abusive husband. To compound the nightmare, the children, who had witnessed the murder, were placed with the father's family, although they had visited their maternal grandparents regularly since they were born and even had their own rooms in their grandparents' house. In addition to the horrible loss of their daughter, Beth and Alan were deprived of seeing their grandchildren.

What followed was three and a half years of court battles that broke the Graftons' bank account and almost broke their spirits. Beth, 51, was described as "an aging, elderly grandmother" and accused of being manic–depressive. "It was as if they were trying to blame Ellen for the murder, and us for raising her that way," says Beth. The Graftons were eventually awarded custody of the children, but the cost of the battle left them shattered. The stress was so high that Alan had three strokes, although a complete physical the year before Ellen's death had found him to be in great health. He lost his business, and he and Beth spent all their money on attorney fees. Two sons refinanced their own homes to help them out, but Beth and Alan remain thousands of dollars in debt.

Today Beth, Alan, and the grandchildren live on Social Security and the money Beth makes from part-time work; she can't find a good full-time job, and they have no medical insurance. In the evenings Beth does laundry, cooks meals, and reads the mail. There are no more dinners out, and the Graftons rarely see their friends, who have different lifestyles.

And their dreams are gone. "I looked forward to when all my kids were gone," says Beth. "I looked forward to being able to find myself as a person, not as a mother or a grandmother but as Beth. It's like I'm lost again, lost raising children. I miss all the things I thought I would be able to do with my husband. All our dreams were ripped out of our book. The whole chapter of our being adults, friends, and lovers together was ripped out, and we're back to raising kids and school and PTA and cookie sales."

LIFESTYLE CHANGES

Raising a child will change your life at any age, but raising a grandchild will turn it upside down. You are no longer young parents with boundless energy; in fact, you might even be at an age when your body betrays you and your health is questionable. You may find yourself in a web of social workers and lawyers that nothing has prepared you for. Your routine, your finances, your social life, and your family relationships will all change radically once you have grandchildren under your roof. Your dreams are on hold. Sometimes you might not even recognize the life you are living as your own.

When my mother talked about raising Kevin, her one wish was that she had known other grandparents raising grandchildren, that she had known that what she was going through was normal. Not only are the changes, and the feelings that go with them, normal, but they are almost predictable. Some grandparents have it worse than others, but each one has stories you will probably recognize.

Your Work Life Changes

Alice Brody had been a schoolteacher for 29 years. She hoped to make it to 30 years before she retired. When her daughter's drug addiction left her with the care of several young grandchildren, she had to quit working without reaching her goal. After her daughter died, Ivy Johnson had to go back to work at a grocery store in order to supplement the government assistance she got for her grandchildren. And although Victor Lane had retired at 62, he had to go back to work when he found himself with three new mouths to feed. It's not an easy age to find work, so Victor, a police service officer, works nights and sleeps days, driving 30 miles to and from work each day. One grandfather jokes that he'll be working until he's 90.

Every aspect of work, from a thriving career to a well-earned retirement, can become a casualty of a second parenthood. Child care is expensive, and so is raising children. Some grandparents quit work to save on child care; others return to work to afford the kids. Many trade jobs or rearrange their schedules in an attempt to both work and care for young children. A Pennsylvania grandmother gave up a career in office management to drive a school bus so she could be home when her grandson is home.

You may have to change your work routine. Maybe you worked at night but have to switch to daytime. Will your job be flexible? Will they lay you off? Perhaps you have to reenter the work force. Will you find a job? Can you handle it? Sandy Blair was laid off from a corporate job during an economic downturn and has been struggling to find a new job ever since.

"I had 103 applications turned in over two weeks and not one call back," she says. "I even applied as a dishwasher at an old folks' home."

The dilemma of working or not working brings up issues of self-esteem and self-worth for many grandparents, as well as the realities of a more modest income and increased stress.

Your Finances Suffer

You worked your whole life and looked forward to your retirement. You may have pensions, social security payments, and savings you had planned to live on. Then your grandchildren arrived. Now you have to use this money for food, clothes, medical bills, and things for the children. "It seems like I can't save anything," says a Michigan grandmother who remembers when she could spend her money freely. "I don't know when I bought my last outfit. Every time I turn around, she is growing."

Court costs can add to the financial stress of raising grandchildren. Some grandparents have sold their homes and watched their nest eggs empty in the fight to get custody of their grandchildren.

If you are a grandparent who has no savings, you face an even greater challenge. It is a severe financial burden to match a lean fixed income with the "unfixed" cost of raising children. Two grandmothers in my GAP groups each have four grandchildren under the age of eight. They live in one-bedroom apartments and can't afford to move in the near future. One can't afford a car; she walks or takes the bus, towing children to school, the doctor, and the market. The other can't even afford a telephone. For grandparents who are also weathering health problems, the lack of a car or telephone can be a catastrophe.

Your Routine Shifts

You had finally adjusted to living without children in the house. You had your own way of doing things, your own schedule. If you put something down, you knew where it was. Your time was yours to work or not work, see friends, read the paper, take leisurely baths, attend to your hobbies. Now your days have been taken over by diapers, bag lunches, and report cards. While your friends are enjoying the company of adults, you are back to the pediatrician, the zoo, and a string of birthday parties. It's tough to keep the house picked up when you have fingerprints and toys scattered everywhere. And your privacy is shot. You have lost your spontaneity to travel or even to eat out. Your day may start at dawn in the rush to tidy the house, cook breakfast, ship the kids off to school, and get to work yourself. For Grandma, it's a distinct feeling of déjà vu. For Grandpa, who may have seen little of his own children while they were growing up, having kids around for 24 hours a day can be quite a shock. For a single grandparent, it's twice as hard.

I received a letter from a teacher in Massachusetts who is raising her three-year-old grandson alone. She finds it difficult to find time for planning her lessons and grading papers, let alone for herself. "I am mother, father, grandparent, and best friend to this little one," she says. "He is not happy to play by himself while I do my school work. I don't think I'd even have time to attend a support group."

No matter how you make your plans, children change your routine. My mother rearranged her work schedule to minimize the disruptions in her grandson's life. Kevin had had to change schools in order to live with my parents after my sister died. Because his life was already falling apart and any consistency was considered important for him, my mother routinely skipped lunch in order to leave work early and pick him up from the same after-school program he had been in before. A New Hampshire grandmother even left her husband back home and spent eight months in Florida so that her granddaughter wouldn't have to switch schools in the middle of the school year. As a grandparent you make many concessions and sacrifices in your routine and lifestyle for the sake of the children.

Your Social Life Declines

"Our circle of friends has dwindled severely because no one else has children," writes a grandmother in Hawaii. "We don't belong with our old friends, nor do we belong with the young parents of our grandchildren's friends," writes another. "I'm a lot older and a lot wiser parent this time," says a third. "But with the Brownies, the gymnastics, the parents' nights, and the sudden earaches, we've lost our entire circle of friends. Our lives are on hold, indefinitely."[1]

It is a complaint that many grandparents recognize: Your social life and your hobbies decrease when the grandchildren arrive. Longtime

friends are wrapped up in activities they couldn't do when they were raising families; they don't want kids tagging along. Perhaps you live in an
older neighborhood with few children. Your friends may no longer have
childproof homes. "Our friends raised their kids," says one grandmother.
"They don't want hyperactive children in their homes."[2] Even when you
can get together with friends your own age, the cost of baby-sitting is one
more expense on an already stretched budget.

Single grandparents, particularly single grandmothers, may also
struggle with issues of romantic companionship. Many children try to
interfere with these relationships. Children may be insecure about a male
friend getting Grandma's attention because her dating may bring back
memories of their mother giving more attention to men than to them. One
43-year-old woman who is raising her ex-husband's grandchildren wrote,
"My life is on hold because I am never going to find a husband or have a
life of my own till they are grown, and by then I will be well into my 60s."

Your Dreams Disappear

More than your immediate lifestyle changes when the second shift arrives;
your future changes, too. Plans get put on hold, and some dreams disappear altogether. It's another loss in a long line of losses. Jack and Betty
Segal had plans for this time of their lives. Jack would be retired and they
would be out on the road together somewhere—alone. Instead, they are
raising one child of a drug-addicted son and helping a divorced daughter
raise three more. "You love the kids," says Betty. "You just resent the fact
that you can't be doing what you want to be doing."

Emily Petersen didn't have big plans. She's a quiet person who had
looked forward to a tidy home, solitary walks, and presiding over holiday
dinners like a traditional grandma. Instead, she is surrogate mother to an
active grandchild and can hardly find a minute for herself.

"We planned retirement to do what we wanted to do; it was our
time in life," one grandmother told a reporter. "Now we can't even watch
the evening news because that's cartoon time."[3] Resentment. It isn't a
word we traditionally associate with grandchildren. But when your life
changes so radically, it unleashes a torrent of complex and contradictory
emotions.

AN EMOTIONAL ROLLER COASTER

As soon as Mandi Fellowes knew her granddaughter was coming, she got in gear: She talked to an attorney about custody, found a day care center, and turned her study into a little girl's bedroom. When Hannah arrived, she washed her clothes, bought new snow boots, and filled the pantry with healthy kid snacks. But she wasn't prepared for all the emotions that arrived with new responsibility and the loss of freedom. "At 45, I'm suddenly responsible for a three-year-old," she says. "Nobody seems to understand what I'm going through."

Every grandparent I know would understand. On any given day they can go through a full spectrum of feelings: grief and shame for their grown children, love for their grandchildren, fear for a future in which their health and finances may dwindle, resentment at a juvenile court system that treats them with disrespect, anger at losing their dreams at this time of their lives, and guilt for feeling that anger. The rapid shifts of emotion are like a roller coaster. Your life is in constant turmoil. Of course you feel unstable.

How much these feelings shake you will depend on what kind of resources and support you have. A single grandparent has a tougher time dealing with the ups and downs of second parenthood than a married couple, who can rely on each other to shoulder some of the weight. Two people may not reach their wit's end at the same time; a single grandparent may have no one else to turn to. Either way, it is important to look at these feelings, to really feel them, to give yourself time to deal with the issues they represent. The more you bury feelings, the more likely they are to fester inside you, erupting like a volcano when you least expect it. "It seems to take about a year to stop denying that this unexpected role is not a temporary situation," writes a grandmother from Oklahoma. "From my standpoint, we all need to know and understand that the cycle of shock, resentment, loneliness, guilt, and, finally, acceptance is perfectly normal."

Isolation

If there is one theme that runs through every letter, e-mail, and phone call I receive from grandparents, it is isolation. When you parent for the second time, it is a lonely feeling. You feel like you're the only one in the world in this situation. You don't fit in with young parents at school functions, but you don't feel right taking small children to seniors' events. "My husband and I have permanent custody of a four-year-old grandson and find ourselves outcasts in most settings, including visits to the pediatrician," writes one grandmother.

You may also feel alienated from your family and friends. Of course you feel isolated. You *are* isolated. Your world is turned upside down, and not many people can accept your new role. Loneliness and even depression are normal, expected reactions to all this overwhelming change. Seek out others who understand, either in a one-on-one relationship or through a support group. It sounds simple, but it's true: The best antidote to isolation is other people.

Grief

Every grandparent raising a grandchild experiences many losses, as well as the deep grief that comes with them. In some cases it is the death of your own child, your grandchild's parent. Your grandchild is a constant reminder of that loss. One grandfather says that the sight of his grandchild always reminds him that his son is dead. "It's a painful thing to live with," he says. In other cases the parent can't parent. This brings a different kind of grief. This adult is not the child you raised. You have lost the bright child with unlimited potential; you have lost the faith that your child would someday be a good parent and a productive adult.

In a sense, you also lose the special relationship with your grandchildren that makes grandparenting so wonderful: the visits, the spoiling, the special treats, the grandparent–grandchild conspiracies. You may feel cheated out of your grandparent role and mourn its loss.

Grandparents whose adult children have died can find solid support and understanding through Compassionate Friends, a national organization for parents who have lost a child. We have also had grandparents and grandchildren benefit from counseling or from bereavement groups, that is, short-term counseling groups that deal specifically with the phases of loss and how to deal with grief. Ask your local hospital or hospice for a referral; social workers, attorneys, doctors, outpatient clinics, and senior centers may also keep referral lists. Understand that anniversaries and holidays will be emotional times for you, and be on guard against plummeting depression. You need time to grieve, and it is understandable that you might want to grieve in private. However, some people progressively isolate themselves under the weight of depression, and then they can't pull themselves back up. If you can't reach out to people, at least don't push them away. You need loving support to withstand this loss.

It is almost easier to discuss grief when an adult child has died. Grandparents who have lost a child to drugs or mental illness yo-yo back and forth from grief to hope and back again. Here, too, support groups can be helpful. Even if your child is living, allow yourself to grieve. Make room for it. You too are suffering severe loss—the loss of your dreams for your adult child, of your relationship with that child, of your lifestyle, and of your grandparent role.

Anger and Guilt

Anger and guilt are familiar companions to many second-time parents. Anger at fate. Anger at the courts and the bureaucracy, which make you feel victimized and penalized for taking responsibility for your grandchildren, especially when you have exhausted your savings and your energy. Anger at your adult child for putting you in this situation. "I could beat that woman for days for what she did to that baby!" said Anne Sutter, whose daughter gave birth to a drug-exposed child and then abandoned him.

You may even get angry at your grandchildren, who are the real victims but who are also the ones who have changed your life. Even when you know that it is not the children's fault, you may still feel resentment—and then guilt for feeling it. "You feel this hostility," says Fay Strassburger, "You feel this frustration. You lose your identity. What are you going to do with these kids? And, then, when they look up at you, you say, 'God, just let me get through another day because they really need me.' "[4]

Lucy Davis is raising her son's daughter, Lindsey. Her son and his girlfriend were both teenagers and drug addicts when Lindsey was born. Lucy took the baby when the mother lost custody for child abuse. Like many grandparents, she thought this would be temporary; she thought that losing custody would scare the parents into shape and that her own life would go back to normal. When that didn't happen, she adopted the child. She loves her completely, but sometimes the frustration is overwhelming: "I should just have to come home and make my bed, and the house should look the way I left it. But it doesn't. There are Barbie dolls everywhere. There's a toy room to be picked up. There's all her laundry to be done. Her dentist appointments. Her eye appointments. She takes up a tremendous part of my time. You can't just call me for drinks; I have Lindsey. I get angry about it inside, although I don't want to show it. But then when she comes in and breaks a lamp, I'm really angry. And I feel so guilty."

It is okay to feel angry. Your life has been disrupted, and it is normal to resent it. What you don't want to do is take out those feelings on your grandchild. One way to defuse your anger is to write it down. Keep a journal or diary, or write a letter to the child's parents—even if you can't (or wouldn't) send it. Just getting your feelings out on paper can help. Find people who can be a sounding board for your feelings. But don't wait for a crisis to call them; call *before* you reach the end of your rope.

Fear

Grandparents who parent live in a kind of low-grade constant fear, haunted by the courts, the parents, their own health issues, and the steady march of time. Not only are they struggling with severe changes to their lives, but they are often battling the normal aging process, if not illnesses like diabetes, arthritis, cataracts, heart problems, and cancer. The questions buzz around them like mosquitoes: "What if something happens to me? Who will raise these children?" "What if the parents resurface?" "What if the system lets the parents take the kids before they are able to care for them?" "How will my grandchildren turn out?" "What effect will all this have on them?" The hard part about these fears is that they represent real possibilities. Parents do resurface. Courts do give them priority. Grandparents do get sick and die. And the reality is that many of these children could end up in foster care, separated from siblings, despite every effort to keep them together. A grandmother in one of my GAP groups died of breast cancer, and now the family is struggling over her two grandchildren; her other children don't want them, and their mother is still on drugs.

There is not much you can do about these fears. You have to look at them head on. It doesn't help to put them aside to deal with later—

although you may do that for a while. Eventually, however, you need to plan for what you can affect and, as painful as it is, accept what you cannot change. If you have legal guardianship through probate court or have adopted the children, you can, and should, make clear plans about who will take them if something happens to you. If you don't have that legal protection, then child protective services and dependency court may end up making those kinds of decisions. But living in fear won't prevent it from happening. Although you can't erase your fears, try not to let them overwhelm you.

Doubt

Emily Petersen sometimes wonders if she did the right thing by taking her granddaughter Amanda, or if she would have been better off adopted by younger parents. "Maybe we drown in the love for the child—the fear for the child—that we don't stop to think that maybe a younger family, someone a little more prosperous, might give them a better life," she says, pointing out that as older grandparents she and Carter are often not able to do for Amanda what they would like to do. "Some days I get terribly tired," she says.

Bonnie and Wade Meyers can relate. The two physicians have been juggling two full-time careers, two high-energy grandkids, and an unpredictable adult daughter for close to eight years. The strain is enormous. For a while, these two high-functioning people could barely function; they would just come to group and cry. They haven't given up, but they constantly struggle with whether they are the best people to raise the girls.

Doubt, for many grandparents, is a normal part of raising grandchildren. You think it's not fair to the kids that you can't play ball or roller-skate or do many of the things you did as young parents. You do get tired and stressed. But I feel that in most cases children are still better off with family, if the family is able to provide for them. Whether you have made the best choice for yourself, however, is something only you can know.

■ HOW TO COPE

There is no question that your grandchildren have brought incredible change and challenge into your life. How you approach these changes, and the feelings that accompany them, will determine how well everyone involved is able to adjust. As you move into a life with your grandchild, here are a few key points to remember:

- *Prioritize.* Decide what is most important and handle that first. Do you need to get back to work to pay bills? Then child care is primary. Don't worry about summer child care if it's just January; think about after-school care.
- *Don't just take one day at a time; take one thing at a time.* Get the children ready for school, then make your shopping list and schedule your afternoon. Plan for small increments.
- *Take time for yourself.* Structure your life in a way that works for you; find a routine that gives you downtime. What gives you a little bit of pleasure? What can you do to refuel? Is it a movie? Reading the paper? Make time for it. When you are constantly giving, giving, giving, you aren't taking care of yourself. And if you fall apart, physically or emotionally, there will be no one to take care of those grandchildren, and they could end up in foster care. So treat yourself regularly, even if it is just a quiet bath.
- *Make life easy.* You don't have to have a perfect home. You don't have to cook full meals every night. Try lowering your expectations and lightening your load. It's okay to pop frozen food in the microwave, or even order in from time to time. After all, there are healthy, easy frozen meals out there and even more healthy take-out choices these days. This isn't about home cooking. This is about emotional survival.
- *Set limits with your grandchildren.* You will have less resentment about sacrificing your life if you don't give up every aspect of it. Setting rules and limits, like private time or a regular bedtime (earlier than yours!), will give you a little time here and there for yourself.
- *Ask for help.* Look for *people* support. If you have supportive friends, use them. Also, find other people who have gone through what you are going through. Check with a senior citizens' group, or ask your grandchild's teacher and pediatrician if they know other people in the same situation. It's important to know you're not alone.
- *Get into a support group.* Therapy and support groups are a safe second family. You will be able to talk about your feelings without being judged or criticized. Other grandparents may be able to help you priori-

tize when you just can't think anymore. You may also find resources in a group: a clothing exchange, grandparents who might be home in the afternoon and willing to watch a child for a few hours. Grandparents who have been in the group for a while are often more than willing to give back to someone in a worse predicament. I've even seen grandparent families take in the kids of another grandparent who was sick or dying until permanent arrangements could be made. The fewer resources you have on hand, the more you need to seek outside support. Even if you are well connected in a community, with lots of friends, you can benefit from a support group. The majority of those friends are probably not in the same situation.

• *Consider your religious community.* Many people get strength from their faith. I know a number of grandparents who say that prayer and the support of their church or synagogue can help immensely. Some congregations have even provided material support, like food and baby clothes, to grandparents in emergency situations. Others have created safety nets for grandparent families, offering everything from safe visitation centers (for parental visits) to baby namings and religious ceremonies to families in need.

• *Make clear emergency plans.* What will you do if you get sick? Who will watch the children? And if the worst happens, who will take them? The best way to deal with fears like these is to address them head on. If you have permanent custody, then make a formal plan, include it in your will, and make sure your attorney and/or other family members are aware of your wishes. If you don't have this kind of control, discuss contingency plans with your social worker early on so that you know what might happen if anything happens to you and you can no longer care for the children.

• *Let yourself off the hook.* You need to accept the fact that your adult child's circumstances are not your fault. Your child is making choices, and you have done the most and best with whatever you had. I don't think people intentionally set out to hurt their kids, and when you raised yours, you really thought what you were doing was the best. Understand that your feelings are normal, that you're not alone, and that you will eventually get through this.

• *Focus on the positive.* Keep in mind why you are doing this and what you have accomplished. In spite of all the stress, there are rewards.

MOMENTS OF PURE JOY

Grandparents sacrifice a lot to raise grandchildren, but there are rewards: the relief of knowing that the grandchildren are safe and happy, the wonder of watching them grow, the pride in their accomplishments. Some grandparents say their grandchildren keep them young. Alta Edwards believes her three grandchildren gave her a new lease on life. She had diabetes, arthritis, a bad heart, and high blood pressure, and she weighed 300 pounds. "One morning I woke up and realized I couldn't properly raise a two-year-old flat on my back. It was do or die," she says. "They got me back on my feet."[5]

And there is the love. It is the main reason you took in your grandchildren, and it is your greatest reward for raising them. "Nobody has ever loved me in my life the way she loves me," says Lucy Davis of her granddaughter. "She was singing a song one day, when she was three. She was in her toy room, and she was singing, 'I have a mummy and her name is Grammy!'"

Joan McMillin knows the feeling. She remembers the night her granddaughter hugged her and said, "Granny, you're the only person in the world who really loves me." "I had tears in my eyes," she told a reporter. "There's something positively magical in the hugs and kisses that makes it all worthwhile."[6]

4

Family at Large
YOUR SPOUSE AND OTHER CHILDREN

> You're going to be fighting the battle alone at times. Your friends,
> even your family, will fight you for raising grandchildren. They
> each have their own version of how you should handle the
> situation, and you have to face their advice and their criticism.
> —*Vermont grandmother*

Taking in a grandchild is about family, and the entire family will feel the effects of this new addition. More than your lifestyle changes when you become second-time parents; your marriage and your relationship with your other children may suffer strains you never expected.

ROCKING THE MARRIAGE BOAT

Ivy Johnson's husband left her when the grandchildren arrived. Frank and Gloria Simon fight constantly over their drug-addicted daughter. And my own parents seemed close to divorce on numerous occasions. The burden of raising a child at this stage of life, combined with the loss of or struggles with an adult child (regardless of the reason), often causes deep problems between spouses who have spent most of their lives together.

Marriages that have always been stable start to develop rifts, and marriages that were already strained may split wide open.

Sometimes the issue is grief. Everyone grieves differently, and you expect different things of each other in your grief. My parents didn't have time to mourn the loss of my sister before they took in her son. My mother expressed it all openly: She cried constantly and all but lived at the cemetery when she wasn't working. My father, on the other hand, buried his grief deep inside himself, and my mother would get furious at his apparent lack of understanding. Grief can rock the most stable marriage, even without the extra burden of new children to raise.

Sometimes the issue is jealousy: One grandparent gives more attention to the child than to his or her spouse, who resents the change and may then spend more time away from home, become engrossed in hobbies, or generally keep the family at a distance. Growing anger may spark fights and arguments over seemingly meaningless things. Often it is Grandma who devotes herself to the grandchildren and Grandpa who rebels. Says one grandfather from Ohio, "We get along, no fights, no shouting matches . . . but [the child] has caused a deterioration of our compatibility . . . I feel pretty much ignored."[1]

But grandmothers are not immune from jealousy, as Nancy Harper can confirm. "He probably loves her more than me," she says, referring to her husband and the granddaughter they are raising. "My husband was such a wonderful father, and everything was 'the children.' I thought once they grew up I'd have him all to myself. Then Scott presented us with Marissa, and here we are all over again."

The sudden changes to your lifestyle will certainly challenge a marriage. Financial stress is always hard on a couple, and unexpected children's expenses raise new questions about how to spend money and how to set priorities. Adjustments to work and home routines leave you with little time for yourself, for each other, for all the things you planned. And then there is the disruption to your privacy and sexual intimacy.

Rose and Gerald Avery had been married for 30 years. Ever since their son Richard moved out, they had been peacefully on their own. At the end of a long day their house was a haven of quiet, order, and privacy. They liked it that way. They could walk around the house wearing anything they wanted to; they could be intimate and sexual without fear of being heard. When they welcomed Richard and his two young sons into their home, that peace and privacy disappeared. At the end of the day the house is now riddled with the sounds and signs of children: laughter, arguments, toys on the floor. Gerald's office is now the television room. Even their bedroom isn't their own—the boys always want to be with them. Their new circumstances have taken a toll on the couple's intimacy. Even when the children aren't home, they live with the expectation that they could come home at any moment. "At times, it's like we've lost the house and certain things about each other," says Rose. The result is that Gerald is often angry. "It's like having four kids at home, not two," she adds.

The most constant source of marital conflict, however, is the children—both the adult children and the grandchildren. In both cases the issues are overcompensation and setting limits. Each is a normal issue in childrearing, but having to negotiate these boundaries at a stage in your life when you no longer expect to be rearing your child and expect only to be enjoying your grandchild can wear on you and your marriage.

Children, Big and Small

Many couples can't agree as to when enough is enough when it comes to their adult children. Whether the issue is money, visitation, or kicking them out, they are incapable of presenting a united front. One grandparent tries to take a firm stand and the other undermines it. One grandparent feels misunderstood, the other unsupported. If the conflict escalates enough, talk can turn to separation and divorce. That is what almost happened to Frank and Gloria Simon.

Frank and Gloria took in their grandchildren when their oldest daughter, Cheryl, divorced her abusive husband and lost custody of her little girls because of drug abuse and neglect. When I met this family, Cheryl was living at home again, sleeping all day and making Gloria's life miserable. She was verbally abusive to her children and to her mother in front of the children. She felt that her mother had stolen her daughters. When she was under the influence of drugs, Cheryl became violent: She pulled Gloria's hair, threw her to the ground, knocked out windows. But Frank kept supporting Cheryl, and it took forever for Gloria to put her out of the house.

Frank refused to believe the severity of the problem. He worked all day and wasn't home to witness what his daughter was doing. Besides, Cheryl was "Daddy's little girl," and he wanted to believe everything would work out. He gave her chance after chance, undermining his wife:

Gloria would reach a breaking point and tell Cheryl she couldn't stay with them, and Frank would let her back in. Or Cheryl would break a window to come into the house, and Frank would let her stay. He refused to back Gloria on setting limits of any kind, whether expressed verbally or in written contracts.

The Simons' marriage almost collapsed under the strain. When things were particularly bad, Gloria would pile the children into the car and call me from a pay phone. "I can't stand it anymore," she would say, sobbing. "I'm running away and leaving Frank." She always returned home, but she was stuck in a tough situation. As long as the Simons weren't working together, nothing could change. Then one day Frank himself became the target of Cheryl's anger. It was only when his daughter threw a toaster and hit him in the head that Frank put his foot down and joined Gloria in her insistence that Cheryl move out of their home.

When it comes to the *grandchildren,* two problems typically shake a relationship: first whether to take the children, and then how to raise them. Sometimes a grandmother will leave a marriage to be able to take in and protect a small grandchild. Sometimes a grandfather will leave when the children arrive. Writes a woman from Arizona: "I'm 59 and raised seven of my own children and three grandchildren. My husband left me over this last child after 33 years of marriage, but I can't seem to let [this grandchild] go." Emily and Carter Petersen had their marriage pulled almost to the breaking point when their daughter asked them to take her child. Emily and Carter were already raising their son's baby, and Carter didn't want any more. They got into a huge fight about it. "I told him if we can't take care of two, we're not taking care of one," recalls Emily. "If I can care for another girl's baby, I can certainly take care of my daughter's. If you don't like it, you go," she told him. "But the baby's coming in." Faced with that choice, Carter stayed.

The day-to-day task of raising grandchildren can cause more of a slow wear and tear on a marriage. One grandparent tries to parent, with all the struggle, limit setting, and discipline that parenting entails. Meanwhile, the other one overcompensates for the child's lack of parents and tries to hang on to the role of the sweet, loving grandparent. The result is strife for the grandparents and confused signals for the child.

My parents fought constantly over Kevin, who was not an easy child to raise. My mother overcompensated, giving in to many of Kevin's demands. My father criticized how she handled the child, but he traveled for business and wasn't often there to help. They felt anger and grief; they fought and screamed. There were even horrible scenes over homework. Every night for months my brother and I would take turns dropping in to check on them and to smooth things over.

It's true that every couple has its fights and bones of contention, but by the time you are grandparents you don't expect to be arguing about small children. You don't expect to be fighting about your grandchildren: you expect to be loving them, doting on them, and sending them home. In grandparenting you have regressed, and there is an added layer of frustration about the change. To quote one grandmother: "Fifty percent of my anxiety and stress is the old boy [Grandpa]. He fights everything I do."

Strength in a Common Cause

Not every marriage suffers from the arrival of grandchildren. There are couples who find that the challenge of raising a second family draws them together instead of pulling them apart.

Dave and Milly Walsh are raising four grandchildren, and their disruptive daughter is still in and out of the house. Dave works nights, Milly is at home with the children, and the daughter doesn't contribute a dime. Milly's health isn't great. The couple would love to travel alone for once, just the two of them, but it's not likely to happen soon. They're both exhausted. It's fertile soil for conflict, but they don't feel it. "Our marriage is not a flashy thing," says Milly. "It keeps going on." Humor and a strong sense of purpose keep them going. Says Dave, "Every six months we think, 'What are we doing? We're supposed to be retired!' But we laugh at each other when we're blue. We want to be doing what we're doing. It's not duty; we're bonded to these kids. If anything, it made us stronger. We're doing something together. People tend to drift apart as they get older; we have a common cause. We're channeling our energy into something constructive."

■ HOW TO COPE

How well your marriage survives will depend on how stable it is to start with, how much stress you have to handle, and how committed you and your spouse are to surviving as a couple. The road will be easier, however, if you keep certain things in mind:

- *Talk to each other!* Often, when couples disagree, they shut down and withdraw; then they aren't open to compromise and discussion. Taking on your grandchildren will add new dimensions of stress to your marriage; try to keep the paths of communication open.

- *Create special time for yourself and your spouse.* It is critical that grandparents take time away from the grandchildren; you need this to refuel yourselves and your relationship. You are both losing out on your plans and dreams for this time together. You must make a conscious effort to do things that make you feel good, or they just won't happen. I know it is hard to plan your own activities when you're overwhelmed by three or four needy, active kids; it's hard to think about yourself when you are so exhausted that you collapse in bed at night and hope you don't have to get up. But you have to make the effort. Your health, your sanity, and your marriage could depend on it.

- *Present a unified front to your grandchildren.* It is important not to argue or contradict each other in front of the grandchildren because (1) they already have low self-esteem and feel that everything is their fault and (2) they can manipulate your disagreement to their advantage (children are good at pitting one grandparent against the other to get what they want). When there is an issue to deal with, try to discuss it beforehand, or take a time-out to discuss it. If you are split in your decision, your grandchild may try to play you against each other, which helps neither your decision making nor your relationship.

- *Present a united front to your adult children, too.* They are expert manipulators and know which of you to go to when they want something. Discuss limits and boundaries in advance and then stick to them. (For more on dealing with adult children, see Chapter 5.)

- *Try to keep things in perspective.* It won't make the situation easier, but it can preserve your sense of humor. It also helps when you can lean on each other for support.

SIBLING SUPPORT AND SIBLING RIVALRY: YOUR OTHER CHILDREN

Grace and Marcus Tyler have three grown children. Their only daughter lost custody of her five-year-old son, Jason, because of drugs and neglect, and now they are raising him. Their son Michael, 29, lives out of town with his girlfriend and his daughter. He doesn't see his parents or his nephew often, but he supports their decision to raise Jason. He calls often and takes the boy for occasional weekends. The Tylers' other son, Peter, 25, lives only a few blocks away. In the past, if he didn't see his parents every week, he would at least call two or three times to touch base with them. Now he rarely comes around at all. He says he will help with Jason, but he never does. Moreover, he complains to his brother about their parents' devotion to Jason: "Do you think they would take care of our kids that well? Look at all the attention he's getting. He's spoiled rotten!" "Peter has been jealous from the moment that Jason came into the house," says Grace. "You'd think that he would understand that this is an innocent child who deserves a chance. What are we taking away from a 25-year-old man?"

Two sons, two reactions, and there is nothing surprising about either one. Many lives are touched when a grandchild moves in, and many relationships are disrupted. The other children in your family are not immune to the situation. If they live with you or near you, they may find their own lives altered. Even if they live far away, they may be rocked by unexpected emotions due to this new arrangement. They may be jealous of the drain on your time and attention. They may be afraid of the toll on your health and your marriage. And they may be furious with their sibling for "taking advantage of Mom and Dad." They may even be angry at you for, in their eyes, allowing yourself to be taken advantage of. Some, like Michael, may offer to help out; some may punish you by withholding their support; and others may simply ignore the whole situation, keeping a polite but neutral distance. How your other children choose to handle their feelings will depend on their ages, their circumstances, and their prior relationships with you.

Other Children at Home

Joyce Griffin's children were in their teens when, one at a time, the grandchildren started coming—all from one daughter and all drug exposed. Joyce had already raised five children and had nursed two husbands through injuries and disease. Her other children were not pleased with this new turn of events. "My children thought I was deserving of rest," she says. "They didn't see me starting over raising children, especially drug children." So when the fourth call came, Joyce's oldest son said, "No more." Then he saw the baby, who had been born five weeks early. "When they saw the preemie—how small, how vulnerable she was— then my children became mothers and fathers," says Joyce. "My sons became the fathers to these children; my younger daughter, who is in college, became the mother."

Nancy Harper's daughter, Jennifer, was 16 when little Marissa arrived. Her brother Scott, the baby's father, was 18, and her oldest brother was 22. Jennifer had been the only girl in the family, the light of her mother's life. The baby's arrival was hard for her. Not only was there competition from a needy child in the house, but it seemed as if her life had been taken away: She couldn't run her blow-dryer at night because the baby was sleeping, and she found herself watching her brother's baby daughter while Scott disappeared with his friends. Jennifer was angry at everyone involved. When Nancy asked her to take Marissa for a few hours, her response was, "Why should I, Mom? I'm going out with friends. I didn't have a baby; Scott did. Just because your life stinks, mine won't, too."

Children who still live at home will, of course, be most affected by a grandchild moving in. Like you, they will find their routine and their living space disrupted by the new addition to the family. They may be asked to share their rooms, to limit their activities, and, if they're old enough, to watch a niece or nephew when you need a break. Unlike you, they had no choice in the matter. From their perspective, a new child arrived and began to take over. A child living at home may feel lost amid all these changes. If, like Jennifer, the child has been the baby of the family, she may feel displaced by this new arrival. Younger children may act out to get more of your time and attention, and even young adults may experience jealousy.

Sometimes feelings of jealousy in your children predate your grandchild's arrival. Marlena Hunt's younger daughter already felt ignored growing up, mostly because she was the "good" kid and Marlena was so caught up with her sister Sharon and her problems. Now Marlena is giving her attention to Sharon's daughter.

Of course, the moments of competition and resentment may be much more sporadic once the novelty passes and everyone settles into a new routine. But when you raise a grandchild as one of your own children, you will always get some sibling rivalry.

When Siblings Are Single Adults

Sandra Cobb has two sons and two daughters. She is raising seven grand-children while their mother is in and out of jail and rehab. Both her sons have been helpful, but her daughter JoAnne has been her right hand. She was 16 when the babies started to arrive and has been like another mother to them, even though the wear and tear on her 65-year-old mother makes her angry. Although JoAnne now has children of her own, she still lives next door and helps out with her nieces and nephews.

My parents were equally lucky. My brother and I were both single adults when my sister died. We had no commitments and no children, and we were already close to our nephew. Like Joyce Griffin's children, Phil and I pitched in, becoming extra parents to Kevin and taking some of the pressure off our parents. No decision was made without us, and Kevin even lived with each of us at one point or another. Even so, we rec-ognized the differences between the way our parents raised Kevin and the way they raised us. We watched our mother overcompensate, and we watched Kevin get away with things that we would never have got-ten away with as children. Phil and I would voice our disapproval and offer suggestions, but these were frequently ignored because my parents thought they were doing the right thing.

Single adults who don't live at home may be less personally affected by your decision to raise a grandchild. Whether they approve of the deci-sion or not, they have the freedom to make their own choices about being involved. Some might even become active aunts and uncles, as JoAnne, Phil, and I did, possibly challenging some parenting techniques, but steadily helping with day care and vacations and acting as parental stand-ins when needed. (My brother even coached Kevin's Little League team.)

Other single adult children, like Grace Tyler's son Peter, may be actively uninvolved. They may vocally disapprove of your choice and may take it out on you by distancing themselves. They may ignore their niece or nephew, neglecting to ask about the child or even send a birthday card. Some may genuinely feel displaced and hurt by the time and attention showered on your grandchild. "But they are adults!" you say in wonder. Yes, but they are still your children.

Many single adults are neither active aunts and uncles nor active critics. These are the neutral ones. They may be caught up with their own lives. They may live far away. They just aren't involved.

When Siblings Are Married with Children

The reactions of married adult children are not very different from those of single adults unless there are other grandchildren in the picture. Then you risk a new kind of sibling rivalry: cousin rivalry.

> "You spend so much energy on Marcia that my kids never see you!"

> "You do so much more for Martin's kids than you ever do for mine."

> "Grandma, how come you buy so many things for Tommy? Don't you love me, too?"

These are the complaints that can break a grandparent's heart. It is hard enough when they come from small grandchildren who don't really understand the situation, but it can be incredibly frustrating when they come from an adult who knows that Marcia, Tommy, and Martin's kids have no one else spending time and money on them. It is particularly painful when, deep down, you know the accusations are true. And it's not fair.

Sue Ellen Rice would love to indulge all her grandchildren, but she is raising two little ones on a meager income. The rest live several states away, and she can't afford to visit them; she can't even afford to send much in the way of presents. It doesn't make her feel like much of a grandma. Ethel Murray's problem is closer to home. Scott, the grandson she is raising, is the same age as his cousin, Aaron, who lives down the street. Aaron sees that Scott gets special things and thinks that Grandma loves him more. Aaron's mother adds to Ethel's guilt with her own complaints. Ethel has explained to Aaron that he has a mommy to buy him things and Scott doesn't. Although she tries to pick up special things for Aaron when she can, the competition between the cousins still disturbs her.

On the other hand, not every married adult child will resent the time and attention spent on a sibling's child. Some will go out of their way to be supportive, including the child in their own family activities and vacations. Sometimes the same sibling who opposed your grandchild's arrival may, like Joyce Griffin's son, become a doting surrogate parent over time. It all depends on the particular relationships in your family.

Remember Nancy Harper's teenage daughter? Jennifer didn't even want to babysit Marissa, but when Jennifer reached adulthood and married, she and her husband offered to lighten Nancy's responsibilities and raise the little girl themselves. Nancy declined. "Marissa has already felt rejection once," she explains. "She's already had one mummy leave her, and this mummy's not going to." Still, Jennifer had made the offer.

■ HOW TO COPE

The preceding vignettes illustrate just a few of the reactions your other children could have to your raising a grandchild. You may find yourself facing completely different ones, depending on your particular circumstances and your relationships with your children. Moreover, each of your children will have his or her own individual approach to handling the feelings involved. However they react, there are a few things you may want to consider in dealing with your other children and as a means of keeping peace in your family:

• *Listen to your other children.* They deserve to have their concerns heard. First of all, their concerns may be valid. Perhaps you *are* overcompensating with your grandchild; you may be hurting her in the process. Perhaps you are neglecting your teenagers; maybe you can arrange some special time together. See if you can find a compromise without sacrificing yourself. Second, the feelings of your other children are valid even if you can't do anything about their concerns. You may not be able to buy *all* your grandchildren new shoes, but you can try to understand how your other children and grandchildren might feel slighted, however illogical their reaction may seem.

• *Validate their feelings.* Everyone reacts differently to crisis, and having your family structure upset is a kind of crisis. It doesn't matter whether your other children are feeling scared about your health, jealous of your time, or sorry for the grandchild you are raising. They are entitled to their feelings, and those feelings are normal. All you can do is try to understand and not take it too personally. You do not, however, have to let them take their disapproval out on you.

• *Don't expect their help.* In your heart you will want the support and assistance of your other children. You can let them know you would appreciate it, but don't expect anything from them. They have a right to their own opinions about the situation, and they have to make their own decisions about how they want to participate. Besides, wouldn't you rather have them help because they want to help?

The situation is different when your other children live at home. It is reasonable to have certain expectations of children who live under your roof. Perhaps everyone in your house shares chores and responsibilities; child care may now be one of those responsibilities. However, try to be sensitive to the needs of your children. You don't want to deprive them of time to do their homework or see their friends.

• *Consider instituting family meetings.* It is easy for members of a family to retire to their own respective corners to nurse their injuries and strengthen their opinions; you could end up as a group of disconnected loners instead of an integrated family. Whether your other children live at home or not, the family meeting can be a way of keeping everyone connected. If your other children feel neglected, you can invite them to participate in certain decisions. If they feel taken advantage of, they can air out their concerns. I can't overemphasize how important communication is in a family, particularly in times of stress.

• *Don't forget your other grandchildren.* It doesn't take much time or money to make a child feel remembered, even in another state. Some grandparents join social networking sites to share news and pictures with distant grandkids. Others make virtual dates through video chat services like Skype, Apple FaceTime, and Google Hangouts. And an old-fashioned greeting card is always a nice surprise in your grandchild's mailbox. Be patient if the other grandchildren need repeated explanations about why Tommy gets more toys. It will take them a while to adjust to the situation, too.

• *Make your own decisions.* It is good to listen to your other adult children and to recognize their concerns, but in the end you have to follow your conscience, particularly when it comes to taking your grandchild. The bottom line is that when the day is over and the lights go out, the decisions you make have to be the ones you can sleep with.

Remember, there are no perfect families, only people who are striving.

5

Your Adult Child

My son has destroyed all of us and is continuing to do so. We just cannot get rid of him. He is just a shell of a person we loved so much. The hurt is in me so deep, and I always ask why.

—Letter from Missouri

She was a beautiful, bright, and gifted child, the oldest of my three children," writes Pam Marshall. "She was reliable, sensitive, and unusually creative. During her grade school years, she never gave us any trouble. She studied hard. She helped her younger sister and brother with their homework. Teachers all loved her. In junior high she started to change." Pam is describing her daughter Linda, and at first it sounds like a typical story of teenage rebellion—loud music, heavy makeup, scant clothing, a little marijuana, and moving out of the house—the kind of thing a lot of adults have experienced and outgrown.

But Linda didn't outgrow it. By age 19, she was using heroin. When her parents offered to get her help, she told them her friends were her family now and walked out of the house. Heroin was replaced by LSD, uppers, downers, cocaine, and crack—anything she could get her hands on. Linda got married twice and divorced twice. She was arrested several times on drug-related charges. At 32 she gave birth to a baby girl in prison. Pam and her husband, Robert, took the infant home from the hospital and have raised her ever since.

Linda's story is not an unusual one. In fact, it is all too usual. It is the story of the troubled adult child, the parent of the child you are raising, the author of the situation you are in. No discussion of grandparents as parents is complete without looking at the adult who is still in the picture.

It is a sad fact, but grandparents who are raising the children of dead or absent parents have a much simpler time of it. Except for the families—and there are some—where grandparents raise grandchildren in cooperation with the parents, adult children seem to have one mission in life: wreaking havoc in your life. For many families it is not the grandchild who is the problem, it is the parent.

A PICTURE OF THE ADULT CHILD

Among the letters I have received is one from a young woman in New York. The picture she paints is a common one: Her mother, a woman in her early 50s, is raising her sister's two toddlers. The sister lives with the mother but doesn't help with the children. She spends any money she has on herself—on drugs, clothing, jewelry, and the boyfriend of the moment. She disappears for days at a time, returning only to pick up her welfare check. "My sister has taken the car and told my mom she's going to the grocery store and doesn't come back for a week," the young woman writes. "My sister abandoned the kids one night to go out with friends." The grandmother has bruises from the children's mother, and her jewelry is gone. She needs financial assistance and custody of the children. She needs to get her daughter out of her house, but she is afraid for the safety of the babies.

Some grandparents call them "deadbeat" moms and dads. These are the parents who show up long enough to make promises, break promises, and disappear again. At best, these parents occasionally visit and indulge their children while you and your spouse play Mom and Dad. Linda brings her daughter presents and tries to be a model mother, but her interest doesn't last long. "My daughter loves her daughter," says Pam. "She wants to hold her, dress her up, play with her . . . like a traditional grandparent who comes for two hours." At worst, they can be verbally and physically abusive to you and their children. I heard from Michigan grandparents who took their grandchildren when one of the men the mother lived with, an ex-convict, was preparing a tattoo for their grandson. Because the mother was overheard threatening to blow up the grandparents' car and apartment, the family fled to another state, from which they notified the authorities that they had left, and why.

Many adult children are manipulative. They may use their children as pawns to extort money, shelter, and transportation from you. And if you have no legal control over your grandchildren, you will probably give in. Grandparents are the first to admit that they have bought more drugs than any other class of people by giving in to their adult children's demands in order to protect their grandchildren.

Your adult child may also steal, both from you and your grandchildren. Just because it hasn't happened yet doesn't mean it won't in the future. Emily and Carter Petersen came home to find their jewelry gone; they had a lock on their bedroom door, but their son and his drug-using friends had cleaned them out. Nor is it uncommon for parents to take their children's welfare or Social Security checks for themselves or to sell their kids' computers for drugs. In fact, I know grandparents who sleep with car keys and wallets under their pillows so that their adult children can't find them.

Some of the mothers are prostitutes, and their parents (with grand-child in tow) may encounter them "working" and then have to handle the grandchild's question, "Isn't that my mom?" Some mothers just keep having babies, who are then taken away because of abuse or neglect. It sounds harsh, but the same stories come up again and again and again. "We're not beating up on parents," explains one grandpa. "We're trying to save the next generation."[1]

The fallout is fierce. Both you and your grandchildren can feel like pawns in a game without rules. The children continuously get sideswiped by conflicting emotions, and so do you. They love their parents and fantasize about living with them yet feel deep rejection, abandonment, and anger. You love your child and hope she will get her act together, yet you hate her for what she's doing to you and her kids. You may experience waves of fear for your grandchildren, suffer guilt that you may be at fault, and spin pipe dreams about the day when your adult child can parent again. Meanwhile, you argue with your spouse and still give your way-ward adult child every opportunity to clean up her act, worrying all the while that the phone will ring one day and it will be the police.

Some grandparents use up all their money and deplete their insurance policies trying to get their children into drug programs. Some pray they'll end up in jail, where they'll at least be safe. Others, less hopeful, take out life insurance policies on their children so that if anything happens, at least they'll have money to bury them.

And then there are the dark wishes and unspeakable thoughts. The thing a parent never expects to feel about a child, namely, that you would all be better off if he or she were dead. "She is 36 years old," says a Texas grandmother of her drug-addicted daughter. "I have honestly wished that she would OD and let her son have half a chance at a normal life." It is a horrible thing to think, but when you reach your wits' end—when the grandkids are in mental chaos and your life feels like an armed camp— the dark thoughts do surface. The painful truth is this: As permanent and terrible a loss as death is, it can seem like a lucky break to grandparents who have to watch their adult children destroy themselves and their families moment by painful moment.

■ HOW TO COPE

Most adult children are constantly in and out of your life, causing continual disruption. Only you can break the cycle, but it takes determination, fortitude, and a few guiding principles:

- *Set firm rules and stand by them.* These parents may look like adults, but sometimes you have to treat them like children. You have to set the same kinds of rules and limits you set with your grandchild, being firm and consistent. You need consequences that are clearly defined, and you need to stand by them. Don't make threats you can't follow through on, or you'll open yourself to endless manipulation. Perhaps you have told your adult son that his friends are not welcome in your house. You may not be willing to kick him out for inviting them over, but you could take his key away. And if despite your warnings you come home and find four of his friends sitting on the couch, watching television and drinking beer, you may have to have the locks changed to follow through on your consequences. But do it. Otherwise, your adult children get the message that even if you talk big, they can still take advantage of you.

- *Learn to say no.* Ruth Castle has a sign on her refrigerator. It says,

"NO is a complete sentence." You have to learn to say no to your adult child for the sake of your grandchild. You cannot give your grandchild a stable home if you and your household are at the beck and call of an unstable parent. Your adult child will ask, plead, and demand all kinds of things from you: "Can I borrow the car?" "Can you lend me $20?" "Can you pay my rent this month?" She will take and take until you have no money left to give, and she will leave you emotionally drained.

Not only is it okay to say no to your adult child, but it is necessary. You will not be abandoning your child; you will be protecting yourself and your grandchildren. Nor do you have to justify yourself. You don't have to give explanations or make speeches. *No* can be a complete sentence.

• *Learn to let go.* You need to come to grips with the fact that you cannot really help or change your adult child. This is probably the hardest reality for a parent to face. No matter what this person has done, he is still your child. You gave birth to him and love him, even if you hate what he does. But you have to let go. "My 18-year-old son was getting caught up in drugs. He's left home because he can't do drugs here. He's homeless, but it was his choice," said one grandmother.[2]

BREAKING THE PATTERN OF ENABLING

"One more chance." It's like the magic ring on the merry-go-round. Adult children beg for it: "Give me one more chance, Mom. I'll get it right this time." Grandparents reach out for it: "She's trying so hard now. If I help her, just this once, maybe she'll make it." Like children on a merry-go-round, they go round and round in circles, trying to catch the magic ring, the one that will make everything better. Unfortunately, there are times when helping someone can actually hurt him, when the chances you give your adult child only allow him to continue destructive—and self-destructive—behavior. In the mental health community this kind of help is called "enabling." When you *enable* your adult child, you are doing more than allowing him to continue his behavior, you are actually assisting him.

Grandparents who enable their adult children often only pour good money after bad. They pay for one drug treatment after another, hoping that each new program will be the one that leads to a cure. Unfortunately, true rehabilitation is rare, and the sad reality is that many addicts don't make it. I have set counseling appointments with many adult children as part of their reunification agreements; most don't show up. Some will clean up their acts for a year, even two years, but then they hit a stress they can't handle and they're back to their old ways. It is true that since I see grandparents in crisis, I don't hear many success stories. But when a person abstains from drug use for one or two years and then relapses, at what point do you trust a success story?

"A sure way to cripple a person is to allow her to sponge off you," says one grandparent. "People who are warm, comfortable, and well fed usually have little motivation to change their lifestyles." At one point Pam Marshall decided to keep Linda away from the baby. "I had to choose," she says. "Either Megan or my daughter. My daughter was an adult. The baby wasn't." But it was still difficult for her. Robert finally had to throw Linda out of the house.

No grandparent gets off this merry-go-round until he or she is good and ready. A support group can give you other people's stories to use as a mirror. It can help you find inner strength to say no and mean it. It can prevent you from spinning in circles as much as you would on your own. But only you know when you're truly tired of chasing chances. Even then, there is that extra inning, that last prayer, that last chance before you call it quits.

When grandparents want to let an adult child come home "one last time," I recommend using a written contract. If the contract is violated, the adult child knows that he has to leave.

Try a Written Contract

Verbal promises are tricky; adult children can claim you never told them something or that they didn't understand. Verbal contracts get renegotiated at each stumbling block and have more holes than a colander. With a written contract, everyone knows where they stand. The conditions and consequences are in black and white. By signing the contract all parties are indicating that they understand and agree to accept the consequences if they violate the terms of the contract.

Creating a written contract is like making a behavior chart or a chore chart for your young grandchild. Your rules must be spelled out in detail (for example, "I cannot sleep until 3:00 P.M.; I must help with the dishes"). It is not enough for a rule to state that the adult child must "find a job in a month." Be specific: "You must not sleep in. You must be actively looking for a job and provide me with a daily list of the employers you have contacted and a copy of the applications you have submitted." Otherwise, your adult child could spend his or her entire day at the movies or online chatting with friends.

Each contract item should have its own consequence, one related to the severity of the problem. For instance, if your daughter runs up a $200 phone bill, you'll turn off the cell phone until the bill is paid back. I know grandparents who took the car back when their son stopped making insurance payments. However, your consequences must be realistic. Try not to threaten your adult child with things that you know in your heart you can't do. If the consequence of stealing from you is moving out within 24 hours, and if you can't bring yourself to enforce that, then your child will have won. She will immediately start to manipulate you and to ignore her commitments to the contract. The purpose of the contract is to provide incentives to change. If you keep threatening to put your son out but you don't follow through, or you let him back two days later, why shouldn't he take $100 from your drawer? Be realistic. What consequences would you really be able to follow through on? Enforcing a contract with your adult child depends entirely on your own ability and willingness to follow through.

Make sure everyone has a copy of the contract. If it is in black and white, no one can misconstrue the rules. Adult children can't say "You never said that" or "I thought you meant such and such." They've read it. They've signed it. There is no gray area. But you must follow through with the consequences or your contract is worth nothing. (See pp. 74–76 for a sample contract.)

Tough Love: One Grandma's Story

"I want my baby to love me. I can't live without my baby," croons Maggie Butler, imitating all the grandparents who can't let go of their adult children. "That's the hook," she says seriously. Maggie knows. She gave her son one last chance to pull himself together, then she finally put him out for good. It was a hard choice. "There is loss there," she admits. "We all lose."

Maggie knew, clearly, that her son's life was in shambles. David was an alcoholic and a drug addict. His marriage had failed years ago, and his two daughters lived in Pittsburgh with his ex-wife and a boyfriend who Maggie suspected was sexually abusing the girls. David had been in and out of detox several times, to no avail, and he had just served two years in prison in West Virginia for assault. But when David's ex-wife abandoned the children on the street one day, he decided to shape up and get custody of his kids. He asked his parents to help him, and they said yes.

Maggie had already done years of work on letting go. She had joined Al-Anon when she finally accepted the fact that David was an addict; she had gone on to participate in other 12-step programs and had used support groups, as well as individual therapy, in her search to understand herself, her son, and the patterns of addiction. "I had already released David and accepted that he's very much on his own," she said. "But, for some reason, I needed to help him one more time. I said to myself that as his mother I would like to see David get his life together and maybe get his children." It turned out to be a costly lesson: expensive, painful, and emotionally draining.

Since the court would not allow the children to live with David yet, the girls were placed in temporary foster care. David came home, but there were strict terms. He had to go to Alcoholics Anonymous meetings, he had to work, and he could not just sit and watch television. "We will help you," Maggie told him, "but you must help yourself. If you mess up, you're out of here." He said, "Mom, I want to change my life."

When David first came home, he was "good as gold." He got a job paying minimum wage, although he had once earned three times that amount. He got his driver's license, insurance, and a bank account. He saved his money and bought a car. He made his parole appointments, and he went to meetings religiously for four months. Then something seemed to change. "I think it was just too much good," Maggie says sadly.

One night Maggie's husband went to a meeting David was supposed to attend. He wasn't there. Later, when her son came home, Maggie asked him how the meeting went. "Great," he told her. She didn't say anything, but she was watchful. She was still hoping he would make it. A few days later he went out and didn't come home. He was gone most of the next day, too. That was the last straw for his mother. As she tells it: "He pulls up at six o'clock like a kid with a hand in the cookie jar. 'I guess I messed up, Mom,' he says. 'I guess I should go in and pack.' I said, 'No, your stuff is packed.' That was the deal."

Five days later, after a three-day cocaine binge, David was arrested for kidnapping, robbery, and assault. He was sentenced to 22 years in prison. He was 26.

Maggie now has her granddaughters living with her. She hasn't spoken to David since then, although he writes to her from jail. She loves David, but she chooses not to be in his life right now. She describes herself as a "hard cookie," but it has been a painful process—a lot of grieving, a lot of crying, a lot of letting go. "I used to pray a lot for David," she says. "Now I pray for myself. David will make his own choices. What I have learned from all these support groups is that we have to allow our children to do what they need to do. They have to make all the mistakes. They have to be the ones to pick themselves up. They have to be the ones to find help for themselves. They will always stay crippled if we are the ones to pick them up.

"I have to give up the control and give him the right to live," says Maggie. "Years ago, I said to him, 'David, when are you going to hit your bottom?' He said, 'Mom, I may not have a bottom.'"

Kicking Out Your Adult Child

Putting your child out is the toughest thing in the world. Maggie had 12 years of self-help groups and therapy behind her, and it was still incredibly painful. Some grandparents can't do it until they reach the end of their rope, and even then they need a lot of support. Everyone's bottom line is different. For the Smiths it might be that their son came out of a drug treatment program and relapsed. But the Joneses may still be trying to help a daughter who has been in 16 drug treatment programs and has stolen the car, the jewelry, and the television. Each grandparent has a different threshold for feeling that he or she has done everything possible. My rock bottom and your rock bottom may be miles apart.

Some grandparents will talk about the same issues for years and still be unable to act on them. A lot depends on how much support you have from friends and family and how much control you have over your grand-children. If you kick out the parents, will they—and can they legally—take the child with them? The answer to that question will affect how long it takes you to kick a parent out of the house.

Even after you hit bottom, the obstacles are tremendous. You may find yourself facing guilt, embarrassment, and your own protective feelings. This is, after all, your baby. You gave life to and raised this child, and even if this is not what you brought her up to be, she is still your kid. You might not like this person, but on some level you do love her. Then there are the fears: "Where will my child be? On a park bench? In a crack house? Will I get a call to identify a body found in an alley someplace?"

You may also confront strong family pressure: relatives who don't approve of or understand your decision; a spouse who isn't supportive and who undermines your efforts; the grandchildren themselves, who won't understand and who may blame you and cry, "Don't kick out my mommy! She has no place to go!"

I have seen grandparents who, with support, have managed to let go. Some, like Maggie, pack up their children's belongings and leave them on the porch. Others give their son or daughter a deadline for getting out. Either way, once you tell a child to leave, watch carefully. You might consider changing the locks in case your child gave copies of the key to friends. Never say, "My child will never do that to me," because you never know. The drugs take control, or friends and lovers exert influence. One couple came home and discovered that their furniture and possessions had been sold. These are things you don't think about until they happen to you.

Some grandparents persuade their children to move out by setting up apartments for them. They may pay just the first month's rent and deposit, or they may go further and pay the rent and utilities and buy the furniture. It's something many grandparents would like to do, if they could afford it. It is one way for grandparents to get a child out of the house and still reassure themselves that he or she is safe. It's a nice idea; unfortunately, I have rarely seen it work. What I have seen, instead, is this: The apartment gets destroyed; the child invites friends over to "party," sells the furniture for drugs, and eventually gets evicted, often leaving the grandparents with financial liability.

Then there are the adult children who won't leave or who leave but won't stay away. You change the locks and come home to find them on the couch eating ice cream and watching television, the window broken behind them. One grandparent had to go through the eviction process with her own daughter because the police would not evict her. And when two Ohio grandparents told their son to move out of their summer house, it mysteriously caught on fire.

If you have legal custody of your grandchildren and the parents pose a threat to you or your grandchild, you may be able to get a temporary restraining order against them. How much good it does is debatable. Dorcas King used one to keep her drug-addicted daughter at least 100 feet from her house. Other grandparents have had less success. One thing is certain. It is difficult to call the police on your own child. But if you must, a restraining order may increase your credibility. Remember, you cannot get a restraining order against a parent who has legal custody.

However, all the techniques in the world will be useless until you are ready to let go.

THE CHALLENGE OF CHANGE

Doug and Jane Sullivan's daughter, Mindy, is 28 years old and mentally unstable. She has three children from three different fathers, and her parents are raising them. She started running away at 13 and lived on the street for years. Her parents don't know if she used drugs. Right now she is living at home, but she interferes with the household more than she helps. Once, when Jane asked her to watch the children for an hour, she came back to a house in shambles. Mindy had put the seven-year-old in charge of the little ones and was lying on the couch watching television. The children adore her, but she can't take them for more than two hours.

Mindy repeatedly has horrendous outbursts. She is abusive to everyone in the house. She gets angry at the younger children and swears she will put them in foster care. She tells them they'll never see Grandma and Grandpa again. Once she actually called the police and said, "I want to get rid of my kids." The whole family tiptoes around her. Mindy orders Doug and Jane around like she's the queen of the house and they're her servants. "We spend all our effort and our money and energy on these children, and she doesn't want to help," says Jane. "Unless you watch it, she takes control of the household."

Jane and Doug have made some progress. They now take the kids and leave when Mindy blows up. She still has her outbursts, but at least the children aren't subjected to her threats. This is not the ideal choice. It basically tells Mindy that she can do what she wants and that her parents will leave instead of making her leave. It enables her to continue with the same behavior. However, it does protect the children from her abuse. Until Doug and Jane are ready and able to have their child move out, avoidance is the best choice they have.

Doug and Jane don't lack resolve as much as they are caught in a complex struggle with change. Throughout this chapter we have talked about changing behavior, saying no, setting limits, and even putting your adult child out of the house. But change is never simple. We always have good reasons to change our actions; less apparent are the good reasons not to. To quote psychologist and author Harriet Goldhor Lerner, PhD, "Change requires courage, but the failure to change does not signify the lack of it."[3] It took a lot of courage for Maggie to kick her son out of her house. But Jane and Doug, and grandparents like them, don't lack courage. They are still weighing the cost between giving in and giving up. There is a clear benefit to setting limits, but there is also a cost. For most grandparents still struggling with these decisions, the issues at stake are love and fear.

When Love Is at Stake

Love is powerful stuff, and Jane and Doug love Mindy. They raised her, they had hopes for her, and they desperately want to see her get better. Like many grandparents, they are not yet ready to let go. No parent wants to give up the hope that one more chance will save a child. Even 15 or 20 chances later, some grandparents are still trying. A family can deal with these issues for 20 years. When you spend a lifetime loving your child, who can say how many chances it takes to let go of her? There is no magic number. It may take two years in a grandparent support group to get one small change in a grandparent's behavior, but that alone can be a significant thing. Remember, each small change builds a path for bigger change. Until you can make larger strides, keep taking whatever steps you can.

When Fear Is at Stake

Fear is also a powerful motivator, and Doug and Jane are afraid of Mindy. They are afraid she could make good on her threats and disappear with the children. She has done it before. Like many grandparents, Doug and Jane have uncertain custody arrangements. Mindy could easily take her children and wander the streets with them. The grandparents would have nothing to say about it. The only way they can protect their grandchildren is to have them in their home, which means having Mindy there, too. They put up with the mother's behavior for the sake of the children.

Fear and uncertainty are common problems for grandparents who don't have legal custody. They feel trapped and may give in to all kinds of demands, including extortion or blackmail, to protect their grandchildren. Living without legal custody is like living in an armed camp, always looking over your shoulder; it makes setting limits difficult. If you have this problem, consider what small changes you can make to create pockets of safety for your family. Jane and Doug's leaving with the children when Mindy flies off the handle is their attempt to make the best of a bad situation. Until you are ready or able to make bigger changes, you can only make the best of your situation.

DAMAGE CONTROL: PROTECTING GRANDCHILDREN FROM THEIR PARENTS

As painful as it is for you to witness and suffer the results of your adult child's behavior, it is even harder for your grandchildren. This is, after all, their mother or father, the supposed guardian and architect of their young world. They don't have the age or maturity to judge their parent's behavior; they can only react to it and be shaped by it. Chapter 6 will look at the emotional and behavioral problems your grandchildren may face as a result of their circumstances. Here, however, are a few of the questions and problems you may encounter when your adult child interacts with your grandchildren.

"What Do I Tell the Kids about Their Parents?"

What to tell children and how much to tell them are tough questions for grandparents, and I have heard all kinds of stories about how people have handled this issue. Some grandparents tell the kids that Mom is sick and needs help. Others don't tell them anything, or say they don't know. One grandmother I know tells her grandchildren that Mom and Dad are on vacation whenever the parents land in jail.

I do not advocate lying to children. First of all, they may not believe you. Children pick up on things; they know when secrets are being kept from them. Second, if they do believe you, they will grow up with a distorted view of what life is all about (for example, that it is common to spend a lot of time on vacation). But, more importantly, if you try to protect children by lying to them and they find out the truth, they'll start to wonder what else you're not telling them.

My parents didn't tell Kevin that my sister committed suicide. They told him she died of a breathing sickness. Later they said she died from smoking too much. Kevin accepted their explanations without question, and as he got older, he assumed his mother had died of lung cancer. When he finally did learn the truth, he was angry. "I felt they lied to me," he said years later. He was in his teens by then, but the shadow of the lie still lingered. "I don't trust them the same as I might have if they had told me the truth from the beginning. Even if I might not have understood when I was eight, I still would have preferred to know the truth."

Tell the truth, but tell it in bite-size pieces. Think about the child who is asking. How old is he? How much can he understand? What is it that he really wants to know? For example, when a three-year-old asks where babies come from, he's not asking about sex. He just wants to know if he was hatched from a plant or a person. "You came from Mommy's tummy" is all the answer he needs at the moment. This is a conversation a parent will have again and again, over time, as the child's need and ability to understand increase. The same standard applies to grandchildren's questions about their parents. Children need and deserve the truth but in portions they can handle. The answers will depend on their age and maturity, how much contact they have with the parent, what the relationship is with the parent, and what kinds of questions are being asked.

Kids ask a lot of questions that don't require whole explanations:

"Where is my mom (or dad)?" "Why can't I be with my parents?" "Will I ever live with my parents again?" Many times grandparents have to admit that they don't know where the parent is. If your grandchild sees her mother, you can tell her Mom has some troubles now. You can reassure her that this is not her fault. If the mother hasn't come by in six years and is remarried in another state, you can tell the child that Mommy is living far away and you don't know when she will come to visit.

Again, consider the age of the child. An eight-year-old will understand that Dad is in jail; a three-year-old doesn't know what jail is. You might tell a very young child that Daddy has gone away and we don't know when he'll be back. As the child gets older, she'll understand more. For instance, Pam Marshall's five-year-old granddaughter, Megan, knows that her mother uses drugs and that drugs make you sick. She knows that Linda's boyfriend hits her, and that's why she isn't allowed to see her mother when he's around. Essentially, she knows enough to understand why she can't do certain things, and in terms that a five-year-old can understand. "We only answer the questions she asks," says her grandmother. "We try to be as honest as we can without burdening too much."

Tell children in pieces, but tell them the truth. They eventually find out, anyway. Children sense a lot of things that they may not be able to verbalize. And be as gentle as possible. These children already have a profound sense of loss, abandonment, and rejection; you don't want to add to that.

"What Do I Do When Parents Lie and Make Empty Promises?"

Jay and Brenda Saunders are raising their grandson Anthony. Their daughter, Eva, has been abusing cocaine for 25 years. At 40 she is uneducated and homeless; her parents fear she may be selling drugs. Eva loves her child dearly, says Brenda, but cannot care for him. "It's a crazy, immature love," she explains. "A child love."

Six-year-old Anthony only lived with his mother for one year, but he adores her. Eva comes to the house and plays with him. She promises to take him away. Sometimes she promises to visit and never shows up; when this happens, she blames other people for the lapse. She also tells her son that Grandma and Grandpa are the reason they can't be together.

Jay and Brenda want Anthony to know his mother. But whenever he sees her, there is a price to pay afterward in regressive behavior or anger at his grandparents. "When she's at the house, we are invisible," Brenda explains. "You can't believe the difference. But when he's with her . . . it's a disaster later on. I think he's furious at both of us because we're not his mother." And it's clear that Anthony suffers. "He's torn," says Brenda. "It's visible. It looks like he's been ripped apart after his mom was here."

Parents promise things: "I'll take you to live with me." "We'll have a house with a dog." "I'll take you bike riding on Sunday." When parents break promises, you get the fallout. Your grandchildren can't help it; you're an easy target—first, because you're there and the parent often isn't; second, because their feelings about their parents are so conflicted that it is safer to get mad at you.

Broken promises are hard on children, who nevertheless continue to believe in their parents. They wait expectantly for the package or check or for Dad to pick them up at school, and they suffer deeply when nothing happens. Broken promises are equally painful for grandparents, who have to watch their grandchildren suffer each new disappointment as deeply as the first. If you are able to talk to the parents, try to explain the effect of this on the child. Perhaps they can run their plans by you first. If you have legal custody, you can even insist that this happen.

You can also talk to the children. Let them express their feelings about what happens with Mom or Dad. Sometimes they don't want to admit that there's a problem. As they get older, they sometimes come to realize that this is the pattern, that they can't believe what their parents say. Either way, they have strong feelings to express and need safe places to share them. Look to support groups, social workers, and family therapists for feedback about this kind of situation. There is rarely one best way to handle it.

Parents may also lie to their children: "Grandma took you away from me." "Don't listen to Grandpa." "Misbehave with your grandparents, and you can come home." They try to channel their anger and frustration through the children, who don't know whom or what to believe. Lies are even harder for a grandparent to handle. You can't control what a parent tells a child when you're not there, and you don't want to get into debates with your grandchildren about their parents. The best thing you can do is understand the fallout, give the children room to have their reactions, and continue to assure them that they are safe and loved in your home.

Again, if you can prevent the parents from making plans with the child, do; have them make plans with you instead. Tell Mom that you'll be in the park from two to three o'clock, or arrange to meet Dad at the library. If the parents show up, great. If not, you'll be disappointed, but the child won't be devastated.

"What If I Suspect Abuse during Parental Visits?"

Continued abuse is a serious concern for many grandparents. Your grandchild may live with you but still have continued contact with unstable or abusive parents. What you can do about it depends on how much control you have over visitation. If you have legal custody of your grandchild and if visitation is at your discretion, you can insist on supervised visits. On the other hand, if court orders call for unsupervised visits and your grandchild comes home with unexplained bruises, contact your social worker immediately. If you suspect any kind of abuse during visits, at least keep a log of what you see and hear, including pictures if you can. Any documentation you gather could be important if a social worker or court becomes involved (see the "Documentation" section later in this chapter for more details).

WHEN THE PARENT IS IN JAIL OR PRISON

Handling your adult child is somewhat easier when she is incarcerated. As painful as it is, you know your child is relatively safe and you know that, for the moment, she cannot physically disrupt your life or that of your grandchild. But the fact that your child is out of sight does not put her out of mind or out of contact with you. You may get frequent collect calls and letters requesting money for things like soap, shampoo, books, or snacks. She may beg you to visit or to bring the kids to visit. Even at a distance, your child can play on your heartstrings. From the time of arrest to the time of release, you will have to decide how much involvement you and your grandchildren will have with their incarcerated parent. There are no easy answers. You will have to determine what makes sense for your family, bearing in mind that what is good for you may (or may not) be the same as what is good for your grandchildren.

"Should I Attend Court Proceedings?"

If this is a first arrest, if your son or daughter has never been in trouble before, you may feel driven to help in any way you can—especially if your adult child hasn't stolen from you, lied to you, wrecked your credit, or endangered your grandchildren in any way. You might also feel guilty about the incarceration, as if it's somehow your fault, or you may feel ashamed or angry. Such feelings can make it hard to decide how to respond. And, of course, you might also feel compelled to do more if he has clear mental health problems—a history of depression or bipolar disorder, for instance. "It's a cry for help," you might tell yourself. "He needs to be in treatment." And you could be right.

If he does have mental health issues and is self-medicating somehow, you may want the court to know that. A majority of inmates have substance abuse problems, and positive family support during sentencing might influence what happens to him. "Judges are often impressed when they see family involvement," says Mary Weaver, executive director of Friends Outside in Los Angeles County, a nonprofit organization that provides support to inmates and their families.[4] "They know that inmates who have family ties are the most likely to be successful upon release." Appropriate ways to help in the sentencing process include attending court proceedings, gathering letters of support from friends and employers who can attest to your child's positive traits, and asking if he qualifies for alternative sentencing options, such as drug treatment programs in lieu of all or a portion of his sentence. Be sure to let your child's attorney know before you do anything.

However, if this is a fourth or fifth conviction, if your child has been vanishing or stealing from you for years, then you might just be relieved that he's off the streets. You might prefer knowing that he's alive in jail rather than receiving a call from the morgue.

"Do I Maintain Contact with the Incarcerated Parent?"

Whether or not to maintain contact and how to set boundaries are primary questions for grandparents when a parent goes to jail. Do you accept collect calls? Do you send money? Do you arrange for the things she has on her wish list? How do you keep yourself from being manipulated? These are the decisions you will need to make again and again throughout her sentence, and the answers may change according to your feelings, your grandchild's feelings, your adult child's progress, and what you are able to do.

If you are unsure about getting involved, it helps to take a clear look at the situation and ask yourself:

- "How old is my adult child, and how long have I been dealing with his or her behavior?"
- "What has the behavior been? Has he run away, stolen from me, threatened my grandchild's safety or my own? Or has he demonstrated that he is trying to improve himself?"
- "How will it impact my family if I help, or if I don't? And, even if I am not interested in helping him at this point, would it benefit my grandchildren to have some kind of controlled contact with their father or mother?" (See below.)
- "What would help look like? What am I emotionally and financially able to do?"

If, after this self-evaluation, you are still unsure, talking to an outsider, such as a counselor, might be helpful.

If you decide not to maintain contact, be honest and clear. Let her know that you've done all you could to help until now and explain why contact, at this time, won't work for you or your family. Your first concern, after all, is protecting your grandchildren, yourself, and your other family members. You can let your child know what kind of behavior you would need to see in order to trust her again and to reconsider this decision. Perhaps you can establish a future date when you can reassess her progress and revisit the question. This might give her a goal to work toward and cushion any difficult feelings that might arise for you in having to make this choice.

If you do maintain contact, you will need to determine your boundaries and stick with them. You can let your child know that, while you still love her, you can't be a blank check. Let her know what you are willing to do—accept collect calls once a month, for instance; send a specific amount of money three or four times a year; send an occasional gift pack through approved channels (see Appendix A)—and what you are not. For example, you might let your child know that you will read any letters she sends the kids but that if she makes any unrealistic promises, you won't pass them along to your grandchildren. You might also want to determine your phone call budget: not only how many calls you will accept each month, but how long they can be. Collect calls can quickly inflate your phone bill, so decide what you can afford, and remember to set a timer. You can always ease up on your boundaries if and when you feel, over sufficient time, that change is truly taking place.

"Do I Let the Kids Have Contact?"

This may be the hardest question for grandparents. I can't say that every child should visit a parent in prison. Nor can I say that no child should. After all, the goal is not to keep your grandchildren from their parents, but to keep them safe, both physically and emotionally. How that looks will depend on the dynamics of each family. Some children with incarcerated parents may benefit from visiting them as long as they themselves were not victimized by the parent and as long as they receive appropriate support and guidance. Again, that will depend upon the child in question.

If you are considering such a visit, you will want to ask yourself some more questions:

- "How old is my grandchild?"
- "Is he mature enough to understand the situation?"
- "What was his relationship with Mom or Dad before the arrest? Were they connected, or was he neglected and/or abused?"
- "How does he feel about contact? Is he eager to reconnect or afraid of being taken away from me?"

Remember, while you might have lots of good reasons to be angry with your adult child, your grandchild may feel differently. Unless the crime was committed against the child, your grandchild may see his parent as just that, a parent.

If you do decide in favor of visitation, here are a few tips:

- Prepare your grandchild for the visit by talking with him before and after the visit. You can explain that he will probably have to wait in a long line, that a police officer might have to "pat him down," and that he will have to talk with his mother over the phone rather than being able to touch her.

- Explain that Mom (or Dad) is being taken care of (for example, has three meals a day and a bed to sleep in) but that there are differences between life in prison or jail and life on the outside. For example, even though Mom can watch TV, she can't choose what shows to see.
- Consult a therapist or child psychologist to make sure that you handle the situation in an age-appropriate manner and also to discuss any concerns you may have that are particular to the situation. You also may want to do some research as there could be a special program in your community that can help you.

Ultimately, your grandchildren are your true temperature gauge. If they start acting up after a visit, if they have trouble sleeping or exhibit regressive behavior, then you know it may not be the right choice for them, at least not now. You can always revisit the question when they are older or more secure with you. However, it may also be a signal that there are things to be worked through in therapy. They may be acting out feelings they don't have words for.

Upon Release

The picture changes when the adult child is about to be released. Some will ask to come home at that time. If yours does, and you want her to come home, do not send money; send a nonrefundable ticket instead. I have seen several situations in which grandparents sent money for a bus or a train ticket for an adult child to come home. They prepared the grandchild to see the mother or father, and the parent never came. Instead, he or she hooked up with old friends and cashed the ticket in. The child and the grandparents were devastated.

This is exactly what happened to Marta Sobol, a grandmother from Poland. Her oldest daughter, Anna, had been in and out of jail and rehab while Marta raised Anna's eight-year-old son, Christopher. Anna was now in jail again and started to write her mother lengthy letters filled with remorse. She had changed, she said. She wanted to be a good mother;

she wanted to know her child, to be a real parent to him; and she wanted another chance. Marta didn't want to give in, but Christopher, always hopeful, begged his grandmother to give his mother another chance. I talked with Marta for months in GAP meetings, preparing her for the possibility that Anna might be using her again and making empty promises to Christopher. Finally, the time arrived. Marta sent Anna a bus ticket and told her that she and Christopher would be at the station. As soon as she saw her, Marta knew her daughter wasn't serious. After all her repentant letters, Anna had made arrangements to have friends pick her up. "I'm going out for a little while," she told her son. "I'll see you when I get home tonight." The child fell asleep at 10:00 P.M. and woke up again at 2:00 A.M., sobbing because Mom wasn't back yet. She never came back. She ended up back in jail after having seen her son for just 10 minutes at the bus station.

Barbara Douglas had a similar story. Her daughter, Rhonda, had supposedly recovered in jail and wanted a fresh start. Barbara and her husband, offering to give her one more chance to come home, sent a ticket. The day she was released, Rhonda called to say she would be home the next morning, after she went to get her belongings. Barbara said, "Don't go anyplace. Don't pick up anything. We'll buy you new clothes, whatever you need. We'll start you over. Just come home." She didn't want Rhonda to go back to her old place because she knew that Rhonda's friends would get to her and that she wouldn't be strong enough to say, "No, I don't do this anymore." Rhonda didn't listen, and Barbara only heard from her months later, when she was once again in jail. At that point Barbara and her husband filed for guardianship of their grandson.

Some adult children don't even make a pretense of coming home; they go directly to their old neighborhoods and friends. Their parents may not hear from them again until they're back in jail. One day they get another collect call, and the cycle starts again.

Nevertheless, there are those who do change. Some get tired of the lifestyle, others respond favorably to treatment, and still others will credit their children as being their motivation to change. They get involved in Alcoholics Anonymous or some other program and start to put their lives together. But successful rehabilitation depends on a variety of factors, including a willingness to change. While I have seen cases of recovery over the years, there have not been enough for me to want to raise grandparents' hopes. More often, I see adult children make empty promises and revert back to old habits.

Once your adult child is about to be released, you will want to be clear on what kind of help you are willing and able to provide at this juncture. You can be supportive, if you choose, while continuing to set and maintain boundaries. For example, you might tell your adult child that he can't live with you but that you will help him find some alternate housing resources.

Remember, if there is no court order giving you legal custody of your grandchild, either through dependency or guardianship proceedings, a parent may resume custody when he or she is released from prison. If you have concerns about your grandchild and the system is not involved, you might want to consider seeking guardianship while the parent is incarcerated (see Chapter 10).

WHEN A DAUGHTER KEEPS HAVING BABIES

Julia Stone's daughter has already lost custody of four children; now she is pregnant again. "We all think maybe it will go away," Julia says quietly. It's a terrible thing to be a mother with a pregnant daughter and to be praying for a miscarriage. But that seems to be the only thing to do when your daughter keeps having babies—often drug babies—she can't care for. You can't force her to use birth control, and you certainly can't reason with her. Yet there are grandparents who are raising as many as six or seven children from the same mother. The babies are all medically fragile, and they just seem to keep coming—partly because the mothers know Grandma will care for them and partly because the mothers don't think about it at all.

The young women who have baby after baby aren't thinking about repercussions or about the fact that they already have five drug-addicted children out there. They are thinking about immediate gratification: the next man, the next fix. Often they are prostituting themselves without precautions. They could get an IUD or contraceptive implant, but they aren't able to plan ahead or follow through. Marlena Hunt's daughter scheduled an appointment for a tubal ligation but was back in jail before she could make the visit. Sandra Cobb's daughter planned to have her tubes tied after her sixth pregnancy, but she delivered in a Catholic hospital and they wouldn't perform the surgery. Before she could get around to it, she was pregnant again.

Even the ones who may not be on drugs but who may be mentally unstable are not thinking about birth control. Liz Andersson's family has a history of mental illness, and her daughter inherited the problem. She is not responsible enough to take birth control measures, won't do a tubal ligation, and has already had five sons, ranging in age from 12 years to 18 months. Liz, who is 65, is raising them all.

Some women seem to have children just for the welfare check. I know there are many parents with large families who live just below the poverty level; that doesn't mean they are using drugs or neglecting their children. The parents I'm referring to are the ones who keep having kids but don't parent them. Often there are drugs involved. These are the mothers whose parents are already raising two or three of their children. If the grandparents get government aid for the children, the daughter may have her "own" baby to get welfare. Women who prostitute themselves for drug money may also get pregnant. If the choice is between paying for an abortion or getting welfare benefits during and after the pregnancy, they may have (and keep) the baby—until this one, too, gets removed by the courts. In the mind of a drug-addicted mother, a baby may mean easy cash for drugs.

Some mothers are even self-righteous about their children. One young woman I heard about had seven children taken away from her by the system before she was 30. The last one was removed when she threatened to push him in front of a truck—and she is sure the system is at fault!

Unfortunately, there isn't much you can do when a daughter keeps having babies. The options aren't encouraging. You can keep taking them, although your finances and energy may already be stressed to the limit. You can try to encourage her to get her tubes tied or get a contraceptive implant, but it must be her choice. Or you can let the next one go into foster care. Wanda Davis is one grandmother who managed to make that decision. She only has one of her four grandchildren, her sister is raising one, and two more are in the foster care system. Diane Snyder also has one grandchild, her sister has another, one was put up for adoption, and Mom has the fourth. Still, as much as you tell yourself you won't take the next one, when that baby comes, it's hard. Sandra Cobb has said that many times; she is now 67 years old and is raising seven grandchildren from the same daughter, ranging in age from 2 to 14 years.

Nor is it always your own heartstrings that get yanked on. Sam and Rita Burton were comfortably raising one granddaughter and didn't want to take in another, but they did. Then, three years later, Mom had a third baby. This time they were prepared to say no. But 10-year-old Tami wasn't. "Poppa, Nanna, you have to take him," she told them. "He's part of our litter." They are now raising the baby boy as well.

One thing you can do is realize that you have no control over your daughter and make peace with what you will or will not do when the next baby arrives. Be realistic about your circumstances and your ability to say no. Your decision is not just about what is best for that baby but what is best for the children you already have and what is best for you. Remember, if you don't protect yourself, you can't protect even one grandchild. Consider what decisions you can live with and make peace with them.

When Mom Has Another Child and Keeps It

There are a number of reactions your grandchildren could have if their mother keeps the next baby; these depend on their age and the degree of contact they have with her. Two common reactions, however, are abandonment and relief.

A child who wants to be with his mother can be totally devastated if Mom has another baby. Feelings of low self-esteem and abandonment are compounded, and the child may wonder, "Why is she having another baby if I'm already here? If she can take care of a baby, why isn't she taking care of me?" He may lash out in anger and may regress to bed-wetting, thumb sucking, and using baby talk in an effort to become a baby again so Mom will take care of him. Older children may simply shut down or break down. Cindy and Jack Stewart adopted Jack's niece Lacey when she was seven years old. Four years later, his sister Helen had another child and kept her. Lacey wants nothing to do with her birth mother or baby sister. It makes it tough for Jack to have any kind of relationship with his own sister because it is so upsetting to Lacey.

On the other hand, a child who is secure with Grandma and Grandpa might be relieved that Mom has another baby. She may think, "Maybe now Mom will leave me alone." The child may, in fact, feel guilt or anxiety about being safe with you while the new baby is with her mother. A child who is well settled with you might be afraid of being taken away. Unfortunately, you can never guarantee children that they will never be removed, unless you have adopted them. Even legal guardianship can be revoked.

DOCUMENTATION

Emily Petersen saved everything connected with her granddaughter— pictures, letters, birthday cards—because she thought she might need it someday. Lucy Davis kept a notebook documenting every visit with her daughter-in-law, whether it was good, bad, or even a no-show. She wrote down everything that happened and her granddaughter's reactions to each event. She knew that her memory alone would not be enough if she wanted to recount these things later on. Each of these grandmothers came to bless her foresight.

When Emily's granddaughter Amanda was three years old, the child's mother (Emily's daughter-in-law) asked Emily and Carter to adopt her. Sheila became less cooperative, however, as the adoption proceeded and told the social worker handling the case that neither she nor her parents were ever allowed to see Amanda. It wasn't true, and Emily could prove it. She had cards and letters from Sheila thanking her for watching Amanda and for letting her see her child, as well as photos of the other grandparents at the house for Easter. Her careful documentation put Sheila's accusations in perspective.

Lucy, on the other hand, found herself facing an angry judge. Lucy had canceled visitation one afternoon because Lindsey started vomiting when she heard she had to see her mother. "Who do you think you are?" demanded the judge, who assumed she was arbitrarily refusing parental visits. "Here," Lucy said, pulling out her notebooks. "It is all here. She had 32 scheduled visits; she showed up for 12." The judge agreed that visitation had to be consistent or not at all and ordered that future visits be held at the child welfare office in order to monitor the mother's attendance.

Even if you're not currently involved with the system, document everything. If at some point in the future you do find yourself involved with the court or even a private attorney, you may have less of an ordeal if you have records of the parents' behavior and the children's reactions to parental visits. You look more organized and accurate if you have information written down in concrete detail and chronological order. If you have to rely on your memory, your statement to the judge may go something like this: "My daughter drops by unexpectedly and intoxicated. The last visit was maybe six or ten weeks ago." Compare that statement with: "On June 14, my daughter appeared at my door unannounced. She was staggering and slurring her speech." It makes a much better impression in court, and you don't have to rely on your own memory.

How to Document

• Keep a journal or log. Use a bound diary or calendar, and keep a daily record of your adult child's behavior and anything pertaining to your grandchildren. Don't use a loose-leaf notebook or a computer log; a bound book is a much more convincing document because the chronological order cannot be altered.

• Don't write down what you *think* is happening, only what you can verify with dates, times, and photos. It is one thing to say, "My daughter never visits when she promises to." It is another to say, "On May sixth my daughter said she would come for a visit on May seventh; that was six weeks ago, and we haven't heard from her since"—especially when you have the calendar entries to prove it.

• Write down everything concerning the parent: the time, day, and nature of phone calls and visits; the child's behavior and reactions before, during, and after the call or visit; and the behavior of the parent. Does the parent appear to be in control or under the influence of something when he calls or comes by? Does the parent ask about the child when he calls? How often does the parent call? Does he visit as promised? Does the parent make promises that aren't kept—ice cream, toys, birthday presents, trips? Write it all down.

• Document what the parent *doesn't* do: when she doesn't visit, doesn't show, doesn't call, doesn't send a card for a birthday or holiday.

• Record everything you spend on the child and keep receipts. This not only verifies what it costs you to keep the child, but could be used later to prove that Mom and Dad are not supporting him.

• Document everything that might be helpful to show a court that the parent is not ready to handle the responsibility of raising a child. If a child comes back from a visit with a parent and has unexplained bruises or resumes bed-wetting or thumb sucking after being with Mom or Dad, write it down. Write everything down.

• Be forewarned: having documentation won't guarantee a positive court response. I know grandparents who had everything written down but were not permitted to enter their journals as evidence, and I know grandparents whose records, though presented to the court, didn't help. Still, it is better to have records and not be able to use them than to need records and not have them. And if you do get the opportunity to present information, you will look more organized and believable if everything is documented.

Sample Written Contract

The Story

Donna and Hal Smith are raising two grandsons. Their daughter Caroline is 31 years old, divorced, and drug addicted. She has been through numerous drug treatment programs, and she has been in jail several times. Each time she is released, she makes and then breaks the same promises. She has stolen her mother's jewelry and even her kids' piggy bank to buy more drugs. Now she is coming out of rehab again, and her parents want to give her one last chance for the sake of the children. This time, however, they are using a written contract, signed by Caroline and witnessed by their family therapist.

The Contract

Rules of the House

Between Donna and Hal Smith and Caroline Black.

The purpose of this contract is so that we can all live peacefully under the same roof and know what our expectations are of each other.

For Caroline Black to continue to live with Donna and Hal Smith, the following rules must apply. These are not in order of importance.

1. Caroline must strive to lead a sober and productive life. She must prove to her parents that she can be a good mother and a safe provider for her children. She is not to socialize with any of her old friends from the street or communicate with them, either by phone or through any digital medium.

2. Our home phone number is only to be given out for employment and emergency purposes. Donna or Hal will take all calls. Caroline may use the home phone only with permission from Donna or Hal.

3. Donna and Hal will pay for Caroline's cell phone provided that they have access to what calls and texts have been made and to whom. Caroline also agrees to text Donna or Hal any time she changes locations.

4. Caroline must be in this residence by 10:30 P.M. and call or text by 10:00 P.M. if she can't make it on time. She is not to be in the house alone, unless given permission by Donna or Hal. Caroline is not allowed to take any property from this residence unless given permission by Donna or Hal. Caroline shall not give out this address to anyone (unless it pertains to a job). The doors of the house and garage are to be kept locked at all times. Electricity and water are to be used only as needed.

5. Caroline is to start an outpatient drug program immediately. She is expected to comply with any drug testing required by her parole officer or by Donna or Hal. Caroline must also start a counseling program to help begin a new relationship with her children. These counseling sessions must be attended weekly. Alcoholics Anonymous or Narcotics Anonymous programs must be attended three times a week.

6. Caroline is expected to find a job as soon as possible. She may not sleep in. She must be actively looking for a job and must provide her parents with copies of her applications and queries to prospective employers. Once she has a job, she must then contribute to the expenses of running the house. This includes food and utilities.

7. Donna and Hal are to provide computer access to Caroline for the purpose of her job search and preapproved entertainment options. The computer will be used in the living room or dining room only, and

(cont.)

Sample Written Contract (*cont.*)

Caroline agrees to maintain only one e-mail address with a shared password. She also agrees to stay off public bulletin boards.

8. Donna and Hal are to provide food and shelter to Caroline. They will give Caroline a bus pass, but they will not give Caroline any money. Donna and Hal are not responsible for Caroline's transportation.

9. Caroline must share in household responsibilities. She must cook dinner three times a week and do dishes on the other nights. She must do her children's laundry, pack their school lunches, and keep her own room clean.

10. Caroline must not upset her children. She must realize that her children come first, and she may not raise her voice or spank them. She is not to make promises to her children or plans without discussing them with Donna or Hal first. She may not take the children away from the house without supervision or permission.

11. At any time, Donna and Hal have the right to ask Caroline to leave if they think she is under the influence of any drug or alcohol.

12. Caroline must leave this residence if any of these rules are broken. Caroline must also leave if she cannot live by the rules of this contract. This is a firm contract between Donna and Hal Smith and Caroline Black. The purpose of this contract is to restore Donna and Hal's trust in Caroline Black and to assure the safety of Caroline's children.

13. At the advice of Donna's counselor, Martha Steven, Donna and Hal must keep this contract in force.

(Date)   _____ Caroline Black

           _____ Donna Smith

           _____ Hal Smith

witnessed by _____ Martha Steven

A reminder: This is only a sample contract. Your own contract should reflect your own needs and purpose. However, try to write it with tight rules and specific expectations. Then, as trust is restored, you can loosen up a little. It is much more difficult to start loose and then have to tighten the rules later on.

6

Your Troubled Grandchild

You raise your kids; you think it's over. No one tells us it's just
the beginning.

—Colorado grandmother

One morning when John and Carol Waters's daughter didn't answer the phone, John crawled in her window and found her dead in her bed with her three-year-old son in her arms. The little boy was desperately trying to wake his mother, who had died of a heart attack in her sleep. When I first met this family, Brian was so insecure he could not let Grandma sit in a chair beside him; he had to sit in her lap and would have crawled inside her if he could have. Grandma couldn't be out of his sight even to go to the bathroom. She had to sleep in his room. Brian couldn't sleep through the night and was constantly telling Grandma not to close her eyes. He was afraid that if she fell asleep, she, like his mother, would never wake up.

Carolyn Parker's grandson, Eric, had been living on the streets with his drug-addicted teenage mother. One day the young woman left the little boy alone in a motel room, and neighbors called child protective services, who called Carolyn. He was like "a wild animal" when he arrived, says Carolyn. At two years old the child could barely talk; he only cried and screamed. He didn't know how to sit down and eat properly, and he was painfully insecure; he hoarded food and screamed every time anyone tried to take his new coat away. "He thought he wouldn't get it back," says Carolyn. "He had nothing he could call his."

Four-year-old Heather Pierce was a very sad, frightened little girl when she arrived at her grandmother's house. She wet her bed, she hid under the cushions on the couch, and she had trouble sleeping. But she wasn't afraid of the dark. Instead, she was afraid of the light. She needed everything shut and tightly closed—the windows, the blinds, the door—and complete darkness before she could fall asleep at night. She was afraid that her father, who was in prison for murdering her mother, would come and get her, too.

Not only are you raising a child you never planned for, you may be raising a child with multiple problems. Many of these children are the walking wounded. They are good kids, but they have not had a good start in life. They may be anxious and insecure. Since the people who were supposed to nurture them have, through choice or accident, left them, they may have a tough time trusting anyone or anything. Many have been left alone in motels and in strangers' homes. They may be used to falling asleep in one place and waking up somewhere else. They have no sense of stability.

Some of the children will defy authority. Some have been responsible for themselves since they were five or six years old. They may have cared for infant siblings, diapering and feeding them; they may have cared for drug-addicted parents. They think they can come and go as they please. Far from being grateful, these kids may resent your taking on the role of parent and may rebel when you set rules.

Some grandchildren are physically and verbally aggressive—with you, other adults, and other children. They only know how to get negative attention and may fight, swear, lie, and even commit petty crimes to get noticed. They will push your limits to see how far they can go until you finally push them away. Since everyone else has abandoned them, they reason, it's only a matter of time before you do, too. Children who have been molested may act out sexually, and even very young children will pick up inappropriate sexual behavior if they have been exposed to pornography or have seen their mothers with various men.

On the other hand, your grandchildren might be the best-behaved youngsters, sturdy little ones who seem to have it all together. You may even count on them to help you with their younger siblings. But an excessively mature and obedient child is also a source of worry. For healthy, normal development, children need their childhood, and that means acting like children. Some of these children may also withdraw and get depressed. They turn their feelings inward and become introspective and shy, isolating themselves from adults and peers. They're your "easy" kids. But don't let this behavior fool you; they may be just as needy as children who overtly act out.

The tricky thing in all of this is that three children who have had the same neglectful upbringing or the same traumatic loss could react in three completely different ways.

WHAT YOUR GRANDCHILD IS FEELING

To understand your grandchild's behavior, it helps to understand what he or she is going through. In the turmoil of a shattered family, children are the most affected and the least prepared to understand or talk about it. A small child can't turn around and say, "I am angry because my mother abandoned me, and I'm afraid it might be my fault." Instead, she may act out her feelings. She may become aggressive at school or depressed and withdrawn; she may have difficulty sleeping, wet her bed, or revert to baby talk. The types of emotional problems a child experiences and their severity will depend on the individual child, on how much trauma she survived, and on the child's age and stage of development when she moves in with you. However, most grandchildren will experience a similar set of intense, overlapping feelings.

Grief and Abandonment

Every case of grandparents raising grandchildren is somehow about loss—for the grandparent and the grandchild. And where there is loss, grief inevitably follows. Whether a parent is absent owing to death or drugs, these children suffer a profound sense of loss, abandonment, and rejection.

Don't let appearances fool you. Children grieve differently than adults do. They grieve like children. One little boy was four the year his father left and his mother died. When his grandmother took him in, he was "a little wildcat." "He suffered a tremendous amount of losses," she says. "Grief in a child is anger."[1]

Nightmares, confusion, and even moments of forgetfulness and joy are also part of a child's grieving process. When my sister died, my mother felt that Kevin wasn't grieving the way he should. He wanted to play with his friends, have a good time. He was trying to put his life back together.

Young children don't have the concept that death is really final. They go from periods of sadness and depression to moments when they block things out. They may not remember what has happened. They may focus on things like toys and friends. They may repeatedly ask if or when Mommy is coming back. The biggest difference between the child who has been orphaned and the one who has been abandoned is the answer to that question. For one, it is certain Mommy is not coming back. Understand, however, that it is normal for children to alternate between overt sorrow and happy self-involvement. It may be hard on you to hear your grandchild's laughter if your own child has just died, but your grandchild is processing the death in his own way. Just as you must mourn at your own pace, allow your grandchild to set the pace for his own grieving process.

There are many resources to help children deal with death, as well as wonderful books that are written on a level they can understand. We used several with Kevin when my sister died, and I highly recommend checking some out at the library (see Appendix A, Sources of Additional Support, Our House).

A child who is orphaned loses his parent once, and it is permanent and tragic. A child whose parents are in jail, in rehab, on the street, or just missing harbors a hope of returning to them but in the meantime loses them over and over again as they wander in and out of the child's life. Strange as it may seem, a sudden death may be easier for a child to handle than months or even years of not knowing. It is the difference between a clean break and prolonged uncertainty, and certainty is extremely important to children.

Reassurance, nurturing, and acceptance are what your grandchild needs, as well as consistency and routine. Children need to be reassured that you will not leave them and that they are safe. These children have a low sense of self-esteem and a high sense of self-blame. Do things to shore up your grandchild's self-image; use positive reinforcement and praise. Remind him over and over that you love and accept him. Predict-ability and sameness are also important. Try to maintain a consistent, predictable routine so that your grandchild can begin to trust you and his new environment. It takes a while, but it eventually sinks in.

Guilt

Children feel incredible guilt when a crisis happens in the family and a parent is suddenly absent. The crisis can be a divorce, an arrest, a sui-cide—it doesn't matter. Children have a narrow definition of cause and effect. It is easy for them to believe that the parent would not have left if only they had been "good," if only they had been more helpful, if only they had cleaned their room or finished their dinner. In some distorted way, they blame themselves for their parents' not taking care of them.

The guilt intensifies if a child comes to you from an abusive or neglectful situation. She may feel relieved about being with you and away from her parents, but that same relief feels like a betrayal of her par-ents. And if she has been placed with you over the wishes of her parents, she may feel like a pawn, split down the middle in her loyalties, caught between her love for her parents and her need to be safe with you. Your grandchild may also feel guilty for being a burden in your life, particularly if she is the cause of friction between you and your spouse. Even when there is no friction, a child may feel guilty for changing your life. "Poor Grandma," six-year-old Lindsey told her aunt. "Daddy is always going to parties. Aunt Dawn and Jason are married now, and they go everywhere. And poor Grandma. . . . You know, she's got me, and she never goes anywhere." "It isn't that I say it," says her grandmother, "but the child is not blind."

It is crucial that you help your grandchildren understand that they are not to blame for their parents' absence or the current situation. Again, the key is reassurance and positive reinforcement. You cannot use logic to change children's minds; you can only continually reassure them. Give them affection and frequent praise. One grandmother always looks for something positive to focus on with her hyperactive grandson. Even when he is acting out or misbehaving, she will ask him to take something to the trash for her or to turn on the light; this way she can praise him and con-tinue building his self-esteem.

Anger

Seven-year-old Gabriel is a good kid, but one morning he started throwing things and came after his grandfather with a pipe, saying, "I'm going to kill Grandpa." Yet at the end of the day, he was hugging Grandpa good night. Adam, 15, told his grandmother he would break a window, and he did; he threw his skateboard through it. And four-year-old Monica has started choking cats.

Anger builds up inside children—anger at their parents for not being there or for breaking promises, anger at you for not being their parents, anger at the neglect and abuse they experienced before coming to live with you. They may blame you for sending their parents away (their parents may even tell them that you did). If they had the run of the streets before coming to you, they may also resist your attempts to impose rules, limits, and structure. Very young children lack words and will physically express their feelings, but even older children may act out complex emotions. Grandparents often become the target of the unexpressed anger these children feel, perhaps because the parents are absent or because the children think that if they do express their feelings, their parents will abandon them forever. You're an easy target. Try not to take this personally, however; you are also their lifeline.

Try to direct and channel your grandchild's anger when he gets mad. Help him verbalize his feelings. It is better for a child to say, "I'm mad because my mommy didn't come to see me today and she promised" than for him to hit someone. Let your grandchild know that it is okay to be angry, that you understand that he feels hurt and confused, but that it is not okay to hit or threaten. Teach the child that feelings and actions are different. If he can't verbalize his feelings, let him get the anger out safely on a pillow or punching bag.

An angry child who threatens someone, even if it is with a plastic baseball bat, has reached a crisis point. It doesn't matter whether or not the threat would have been carried out. The fact that the child was that angry and couldn't channel that feeling is a warning sign. Children who have reached this point could hurt someone; they could also hurt themselves. If the problem isn't addressed, it may only worsen as they get older. Anger that is extreme or disrupts your daily life is a sign of crisis. This is the time to seek professional counseling for the child—and for yourself, so that you can learn to help her.

Fear, Anxiety, and Insecurity

Every child has fears of some sort—of the dark, the boogeyman, being lost. The world is a big place full of dangerous unknowns, and children are particularly powerless in it. But while a night-light can take care of a childish fear of the dark and you can talk about the questionable existence of the boogeyman, what can you do about a child who has already lived the nightmare? Your grandchild knows there are real things to fear because she has seen them. The child may not trust adults because her parents proved untrustworthy. She is probably terrified of being abandoned again, this time by you. "Who will take care of me if Grandma gets sick?" is a scary thought for a kid, and "What if Grandma dies?" is even scarier.

When Marilyn McIntosh first got her grandchildren, they were anxious and insecure. They asked questions like these: "Do you love us as much as you loved your own kids?" "Are you and Grandpa always going to live together?" "Are you going to live long enough for me to grow up and take care of myself?"[2] As time passes and children are exposed to the constancy of a loving, safe environment and a normal, predictable daily routine—having their clothes and toys in the same place each day and sleeping in the same bed every night—the questions come less frequently. But they are probably never far from the surface. Anne Sutter was just flopped across her bed one day, tired after a grueling day at work. Perhaps she dozed awhile. It was enough to panic her six-year-old grandson. Anne woke to a child frantically shaking her foot and yelling, "Mommy! I thought you were dead!"

There are also fears about the parents: "Won't they ever come back?" Or the reverse: "What if they *do* come back?" One little boy was so afraid that his mother would come and take him that he built traps for her; he rigged a gate with rubber snakes so that if she tried to open the gate, the snakes would pop up and scare her away.[3]

Reassuring frightened children takes time, patience, and consistency—not just the consistency of reassuring words and hugs but of three meals a day, regular school hours, a stable routine. You will also need clear contingency plans in case of emergency. Even the healthiest grandparents can get sick, and death is an unavoidable fact of life at any age. Seriously consider who will care for your grandchildren if you cannot, make it as formal as your legal situation allows, and when your grandkids are old enough to understand, let them know. Understand that you may have to reassure your grandchildren again and again as they slowly adjust to their new situation. Extreme fears, however, may indicate a need for counseling.

Embarrassment

Some children may be sensitive about the fact that they live with grandparents, particularly when other children are around. They may also be embarrassed by their parents. It is difficult for children to accept the fact that their situation is different from that of their peers. Their friends may ask painful questions and tease them. The parents of their friends are probably younger and able to participate in more activities. Although there are increasing numbers of older first-time parents, as well as young grandparents, the age factor can spark embarrassing, if innocent, questions. "Where's your mother?" a little girl in the playground asked seven-year-old Melissa one day. The little girl had heard Melissa call her 70-year-old grandmother "Mommy" and didn't believe mothers had so much gray hair. "Where's your mother?" the little girl persisted. Melissa didn't know how or what to answer. She doesn't know where her mother is—her mother abandoned her when she was 10 months old and she has never seen her. Grandma overheard the exchange and came to her rescue. "Why do you ask so many questions?" she asked the little girl; then she changed the subject.

Perhaps you live in a small community and your grandchild's friends know that the child's parent is in jail or on drugs. The teasing may be far less innocent. Children can be cruel, and they will use whatever ammunition they can find to inflict pain. Fifteen-year-old Vanessa constantly gets into fights at school. The other children say horrible things to her: that her mother was a "jailbird," that her mother didn't want her, that her mother had syphilis. Vanessa says that she gets into fist fights because the taunts make her "crazy."

Sometimes the parent's presence itself is the problem. Sixteen-year-old Mark remembers coming home from shopping one day to find his mother stretched out on the front lawn looking "like a bum." He recalls, "I felt so embarrassed; I never wanted to come back. My friends were standing around and said, 'Who's that?' I said, 'Just a friend of the family.' I can't believe I said that. And then someone said, 'That's his mother.' Everybody knew about my mother by then, but nobody ever saw her. And she was lying on the grass, and the neighbors were staring."

These are hard situations to face, and there is no perfect way to handle them. Teach your grandchildren that they don't have to answer questions that make them uncomfortable, that they can change the subject or say, "I don't want to talk about that right now." Teach them to use their words, not their fists, when they are angry. But, most importantly, try not to be hurt by their hurt and embarrassment. When they talk about these feelings at home, it is important to listen and acknowledge their pain. Growing up is hard enough without all these extra problems. What they most need is for you to understand that. You can't make it go away and you can't make it better, but you can certainly listen.

Hope and Fantasy

Unless they are terrified of them, your grandchildren will probably never give up the hope, the fantasy, that their parents will someday come back and take care of them. Although they love you, the parent–child bond is a tight one that rarely vanishes—even when a child has been mistreated. Ten-year-old Stephanie was abandoned by her mother when she was two years old. She hasn't seen her in five years, but she still fantasizes about her. One day Stephanie called 911 and asked the sheriff to find her mother. Although five-year-old Marcy was physically and sexually abused, she still talks about going back and living with Mom. Many children want to remain with their grandparents, but they fantasize about having their parents join them. When five-year-old Megan's mother asked Megan if she wanted to live with her, the child replied, "No, I want you to come live with all of us in the same house."

These hopes and fantasies can result in erratic behavior on the part of the child. Some children act out in the hope that their grandparents will be unable to handle them and will send them back to their parents. Others will become depressed and withdrawn. Says one grandmother, "The kids believe their mom will come get them. When it doesn't happen, we get anger." The reverse is also true: Children who are returned to their parents and are unhappy may misbehave so they will be sent back to Grandma's.

It is normal for your grandchildren to have these hopes and dreams and to be disappointed when they don't come true. All you can do is let them know you understand their feelings and that you will continue to be there for them when they need you.

COMMON BEHAVIOR PROBLEMS

Every child who lives with grandparents suffers some part of this emotional kaleidoscope. Children need reassurance that their thoughts and feelings are normal and that most other children in their situation would have similar ones. Encourage your grandchildren to express their feelings in whatever way they can, provided they don't hurt themselves or others in the process. If they can talk about being hurt or angry or frightened, they are less likely to channel those feelings into inappropriate or negative behavior.

Not every child, however, is capable of verbalizing feelings. Sometimes the feelings are too big; sometimes there are too many of them. And many children are too young to understand what they are going through, let alone to talk about it.

What follows are some common behavior problems and parenting issues that trouble grandparents. Remember, children act out what they cannot verbalize. These behavior problems are mostly symptoms of underlying emotional issues. Sometimes several behaviors may be related to one issue. For instance, a child who is experiencing eating and sleeping disorders as well as severe "clinginess" may be suffering from a shattered sense of trust and will need your help to restore it. On the other hand, these three behaviors could have three different emotional roots. In any case, both your grandchild's behavior and the feelings behind it will need to be addressed for the child to make a healthy adjustment to his or her new living situation.

Excessive Clinging

Fear and insecurity can make a grandchild excessively clingy. Carol Waters couldn't take a shower without her grandson Brian in the bathroom. He wanted to sit in her lap in public, not next to her. He didn't want to be left at school or with a baby-sitter and cried excessively when she left.

When their grandparents are attending a GAP session, the children will often wander past the door and peek in just to make sure that Grandma or Grandpa is still in the same place. Five-year-old Megan often sleeps in Grandma's lap through the whole session to avoid having to leave her grandmother and go with the other kids. And one day when six-year-old Gregory saw the group members leave the room and his grandmother was not among them—she was in the bathroom—he let out a bloodcurdling scream: "Where is my grandma!?"

Most children have clingy moments, but for these children clinging is almost a way of life. They may also talk excessively as a way of keeping adults not only physically present but also mentally and emotionally present. For a harried grandparent, behavior like this can be hard to handle. Try to understand that your grandchild doesn't want to drive you crazy but is only trying to stay safe. These children are terrified of being left or forgotten, even for a moment. It takes time, reassurance, and consistency for grandchildren to trust again and feel secure. Once they start trusting that you will continue to be there for them, and can see it with their own eyes, the clingy behavior will ease up (although it may reappear again in times of change).

For severe situations like Brian's, however, therapy may be needed. I worked with Carol Waters's grandson Brian in individual and family therapy for several years. At first I had Grandma stay in the office with us for the entire time. Then I told her to say in the middle of the therapy session that she had to go to the bathroom. Brian would scream and yell in a fit of anger and panic. I would hold him at the door of the bathroom while Carol talked to him from the other side. Then she would be silent for a minute and come out. Brian thought she was going to disappear through some secret door in there. He finally reached the point where he could see me without having Grandma in the room and could go off to play in the park with other children during GAP events. But it took time, patience, and a great deal of consistency and reassurance.

Sleeping Problems

Five-year-old Patrick was raised by a mentally ill mother and an abusive father and stepmother before coming to live with his grandmother. He is so frightened and insecure that he can't sleep in his own room; he sleeps on a mat on the floor by Grandma. The same thing happened with Kevin after my sister died. I had temporarily moved in with my parents after graduate school and slept on a mat on the floor next to Kevin's bed. My nephew wouldn't sleep unless I was holding his hand. If I moved at all, he would wake up instantly. If I wasn't there, he would take his blanket in the middle of the night and lie down beside my parents' bed. He was very afraid that people were going to die on him again, and we were all he had.

Sleeping problems are common with children whose lives have been disrupted. They take the form of nightmares, fear of the dark, and wanting to sleep with the grandparents. These are unspoken cries of insecurity and indicate a need for reassurance, nurturing, and trust.

Going to bed can be a difficult time for your grandchild. It means a long separation from you and may tap fears that you could disappear in the night or that she may wake up in a strange environment. Again, reassurance, consistency, and a predictable routine are key. Try to establish a bedtime ritual. Set a bedtime hour and stick to it. As you tuck your grandchild in, talk about how the day went and any plans you may have for tomorrow, letting her know you will be there if she gets scared at night and when she wakes up in the morning. You can even leave a picture of yourself or the family by the bed to reassure her. Bedtime rituals can be a wonderful, secure part of childhood, a time that your grandchild may use to discuss the day or confide in you.

If, on the other hand, you have a grandchild who can't sleep or wakes up with nightmares, there are a number of things you can try to get him back to bed: You can rub his back, sing to him, or read him bedtime stories to quiet him down (although you don't want to reward waking up if it becomes a nightly habit). A night-light in the room and hallway can help youngsters who have nightmares. Try to address the problem in the child's room. Children need to feel secure in their own beds, and sleeping alone is an important step in learning a healthy autonomy. Besides, you need your privacy, too. Once you consistently allow a child to sleep in your bed, the habit is more difficult to break.

As children begin to work through their fears and rebuild trust, their sleeping problems should start to dissipate. My nephew Kevin eventually learned to sleep alone in his room, and Heather Pierce has begun to sleep with her windows open. But it takes time, patience, and, with some children, counseling to help them process the trauma and loss they have experienced.

Eating Problems

Food can be the focus of several kinds of problems for your grandchildren. They may not have had enough to eat before they came to you. They may eat too fast or too much, as if each meal might be their last for some time. They may even start hoarding food. When two-year-old Eric arrived at his grandparents' house, he ate so quickly he was in danger of choking. "Eric, take little bites; there's plenty of food," his grandmother would assure him. And six-year-old Daryl hides food under his bed, even cans he can't open.

On the other hand, some children may get depressed and stop eating or may refuse to eat, using mealtime as a way to get your attention. Charlotte Buckley has a four-year-old grandson who turns food into a power struggle. Joey won't take a bite unless Grandma is there to bribe and spoon-feed him; sometimes even that doesn't do any good. He does eventually eat, however, when she ignores him.

When you are dealing with a problem concerning food, whether a child is eating too much or too little, you need to rule out any medical problems. Most likely the problem is related to psychological issues, but you don't want to overlook any physical cause.

A change in a child's eating pattern is often a symptom of depression. Consider it in the context of your grandchild's overall behavior: Is there also a change in sleeping pattern? Is the child becoming withdrawn and isolated? If so, you may want to have her evaluated for depression and treated accordingly.

Children who hoard, like Eric and Daryl, need to be reassured that there is plenty of food. They do well with a consistent eating routine. If they know they will have breakfast, lunch, an after-school snack, and dinner at the same time each day, they can start to view meals as something they can count on. If they can tell time, they can see when the next meal will be. Children who eat too fast or too much may need to be monitored for a while. They should be served small portions and encouraged to ask for more if they are still hungry. You might also consider keeping healthy snack foods in a place your grandchildren can reach; this practice will reassure them that if they do get hungry, they can do something about it. It gives them a safe sense of control over their food.

A child like Joey has a different problem. For him, food is a way to manipulate Grandma. Why should he make an effort to eat by himself when refusing to eat earns him Charlotte's undivided attention? If you have a grandchild like Joey, understand that this is a different control issue: It is not about controlling food, it is about controlling you and the environment. If your grandchild can get you to sit in the kitchen for three hours trying to get him to eat, he wins. You can, however, step outside of the power struggle.

Again, the key is firmness, consistency, and patience. Have regular meals that last a usual and reasonable length of time. Let your grandchild know that if she hasn't eaten by the end of the meal, she may have to wait until the next one. Since children have a poor sense of time, it's a good idea to use a timer to let her know when the meal is over. When she realizes she won't have someone sitting and coaxing her to eat—and she misses a meal or two—she'll start eating.

If you do use this technique, you must be consistent. It doesn't do any good if you feel sorry for your grandchild and provide a snack later on. All he will learn is that he can eat whenever, and whatever, he wants. What you can do is remind the child that he can't have a snack today because he didn't eat his dinner, that perhaps if he eats dinner tomorrow, he can also have dessert. Don't forget to check with your pediatrician regarding vitamins and proper nutrients, and, again, make sure the problem isn't medical.

However your grandchild relates to food, never withhold meals as punishment; eating should be a safe and reliable experience for a child, not something to be earned.

Babyish Behavior

Three-year-old Savannah reverts to using diapers and a bottle whenever she sees her mother, although she doesn't use either in nursery school or at home. "I think she thinks Mary wants her to be in diapers and bottles," says her grandmother, who traces Savannah's babyish behavior to the birth of her twin sisters. Ever since that time, Savannah has been possessive of her mother, trying to prevent her from holding the infants.

When young children feel threatened, they may revert to babyish behavior: thumb sucking, baby talk, using a bottle, bed-wetting, clinging, wanting to be carried, or waking up in the middle of the night. A new sibling is certainly a threat. A child may feel insecure because everyone is paying attention to the baby in the family, a position she held until now. She may feel rejected if Mom keeps the new child but doesn't take her. A sibling is not the only threat a child faces; each time she sees a parent leave, it can feel like rejection. If her mother was nurturing during the child's infancy, an insecure six-year-old, hoping to bring Mom back, might revert to babyish behavior.

Understand that these are normal reactions. Most children will regress briefly, and need to, in order to work through changes in their life circumstances. Acting like a baby may be a sign that they need extra nurturing or need to adopt the role of a baby for a while. Eventually, they return to their more mature selves. Some children, however, will cling to this baby identity and not progress to the next stage of development.

If your grandchild is regressing, allow him some room to be a baby and work out the feelings. If the situation doesn't resolve itself, don't let it continue too long. You can address the insecurities without encouraging the babyish behaviors. You can validate the child's feelings with questions like "Do you wish you were still a baby?" or "Do you wish you still had your bottle?" Recognizing and understanding the feelings is different from encouraging the actions. You can reassure your grandchild that you love him and that he is very special but also remind him that he is no longer a baby. You can point out the advantages of being big and the disadvantages of being a baby: Big children can play with toys and watch television; babies take lots of naps and don't get to make decisions. Remind your grandchild to use words, not baby talk. Be reassuring and nurturing but also firm.

One more thing you can do is create a "life book" for your grandchild, that is, a collection of photos from the past arranged in chronological order, like a story, with descriptions underneath each photo. It is important for children to have a sense of roots and progress, and photos clearly document the passage of time. Your grandchild can see herself when she really was little, and she can see how much she has grown. There is a healing power in being able to hold your history in your hand

and look at it, even for a small child. If you want to do a life book for your grandchild and you don't have access to early photos, start with the pictures you have. Add to the life book as often as you can, depending on your time and circumstances. You don't have to wait for major events like birthdays and holidays to take snapshots. Everyday activities can make charming photos and tell a story about a child's life.

Wanting to Call You Mom and Dad

A child who has a relationship with his parents already knows them as Mom and Dad and knows you as Grandma and Grandpa. Other children, however, may want to call you Mom and Dad; all the other kids have mothers and fathers, and your grandchildren don't like feeling different. Older children may even want to have their names changed whereas little ones tend to call anyone who nurtures them "Momma."

The truth is that you will probably have a harder time with this issue than your grandchildren. You may not want the children to forget their parents and may fear that this could erase their memory.

You might feel like you are usurping their parents' place. Or you might just be uncomfortable: You were a parent, now you are a grandparent, and you want the difference to be clear. When the subject of names comes up, don't make it a big emotional issue for a child. It is all individual, and there are no right or wrong answers. Whatever you and your grandchild are comfortable with will probably work fine. If you and your spouse are not comfortable being called Mom and Dad, you can tell your grandchildren that you are doing all the things a parent does but that they still have a mom and a dad and you are Grandma and Grandpa.

"Stuart asks me about how I can be both Grandma and Momma," says Arlene Townsend. "I tell him, 'I am what you want me to be.'" Three-year-old Tamara refused to call her mother "Mommy" when she saw her on visits. Her grandmother asked her why. "Her not my mommy," the little girl replied, "She's just my friend. You're my mommy. You take care of me every day." And Denise, who has lived with her grandparents from the day she was born, has it all squared away: Her grandmother is Grandma, her grandfather is Daddy, her Aunt Carla is Momma, and her mother is Momma Gail.

Tests and Manipulation

All children test limits; it is how they discover the boundaries in their world. They mouth off and act out and then learn from our reactions what is acceptable behavior and what is not. They don't fight fair, either. Children know just what to say, and when to say it, to get you to melt. They use scraped knees and hurt feelings, pouts, whines, and tears to get their way. Some parents handle the tests and manipulations of childhood better than others, but it is all part and parcel of raising kids.

Many grandparents forget this fact. Perhaps you haven't lived with small children in years and have allowed your memories of childrearing to mellow over time. You may be surprised and frustrated when your grandchildren are hard to handle; unfortunately, your grandchildren may be harder to handle than most children their age.

Tragic circumstances have given many grandchildren a distorted sense of limits. If parents were unstable and inconsistent—punishing today behavior they permitted yesterday—your grandchildren may see rules as flexible and changeable. Children who had free reign with their parents may have learned that they can do as they please. They may not think your rules apply to them and may resent your attempts to impose structure on their lives. They will test and retest the limits you set for them, beyond the point where other children would give up. Because these grandchildren struggle with profound feelings of rejection, abandonment, and poor self-esteem, they will also test how far they can go before you, too, reject them. They will push you away before you push them away.

Your grandchildren also have a stronger arsenal than most kids in the "I'm so unhappy; just do it my way" phase of childhood. While the reality of being neglected, abandoned, or abused is tragically painful, it may also be used as a means of manipulating adults. Every child cries "I want my mommy" when someone else—even Daddy—sets limits. (And if Mommy sets limits, "I want my daddy" might do just fine.) But it's a whole new ball of wax when it's a grandchild raised by grandparents. When Mommy might be in jail, on the streets, or even dead, a plaintive "I want my mommy" can just about kill Grandma, and she usually melts.

Don't underestimate the intelligence of children, particularly these kids. Many of them have picked up traits and characteristics from parents who are equally manipulative—addicts are the greatest con artists in the world—and most of these children are smart enough to push your buttons. They play for sympathy. They get Grandma and Grandpa fighting and take advantage of that. They tell their tragic stories to teachers, counselors, and peers as justification for poor behavior or as a means of getting their way. When Kevin was in school, he once tried to get himself out of trouble by telling the teacher his mom had died. I think he believed he wouldn't have to be responsible for his behavior if he drew on something tragic.

Meanwhile, you start the game with your defenses weakened. Your grief at the situation, the split in your identity between grandparent and parent, your need to nurture these children and show them they are loved—all these factors make you vulnerable to manipulative behavior. There is, after all, a fine line between being a doting grandparent and a second-time parent with a need to discipline. Often you slip from one role to the other almost without noticing, and the kids know how to get you to do just that.

■ HOW TO COPE

• *Set a clear, daily routine.* Children need consistency, particularly children who have suffered from loss and uncertainty. Try to make some aspects of your daily life predictable. Have clear expectations for each day, and warn your grandchildren about any expected changes. Recognize that change may trigger a repeat of unwanted behavior.

• *Offer positive choices.* Build regular choices into your grandchild's life. Allow him to have control over which book he reads at night, what stuffed animal he takes to bed, whether he eats his peas or potatoes first at dinner, whether he wears the blue pants or the green ones to school. Let him make decisions about things that don't matter to you or between two equally acceptable choices. Making decisions will give your grandchild a sense of control and may spare him from needing to seek power in negative ways.

• *State rules in the positive.* Whenever possible, tell your grandchildren what you want them to do instead of what you don't want them to do. You don't want to sound like you're constantly criticizing. If children follow positive rules, they feel they are accomplishing something, instead of simply succeeding in avoiding punishment.

• *Set limits and stick to them.* Children need firm, consistent limits. As much as they resist them, limits give children a sense of security and help them know what the expectations are in the world around them.

• *Present a united front.* Divide and conquer is a classic military maneuver, but kids seem to have an instinct for it. Your grandchildren know whom to go to for whatever they want, and they will play one grandparent against the other to get it. Try to make parenting decisions with your spouse, and stick to them. Otherwise, your grandchild may "win," and your marriage may suffer.

• *Learn to recognize manipulation.* One of the biggest problems in handling manipulative behavior is recognizing it, particularly in such troubled children. These children are surviving enormous tragedies, and yet some are arch manipulators. How do you know whether your grandchild is really missing her mother right now or just trying to stay up for another hour (or both, as is often the case)? You will need to rely on your instincts, the advice of counselors, and how well you know this child. Consider these factors: the timing of the outburst, the age of the child, and the child's level of sophistication. Put yourself in the child's place. Why is she doing this? If you have just refused to give the child a candy bar or it is bedtime, she may be trying to push your buttons. It's different when a child scrapes a knee and can't stop crying because Mom, who is no longer here, was most nurturing at such a time.

• *Separate feelings and actions.* Whether a child's tears or bids for sympathy stem from manipulation, emotional turmoil, or a combination of the two, there is one important thing to keep in mind: Feelings and behavior are not the same. It is important to reassure your grandchild that all his feelings are valid. He has a right to be sad or mad or upset. But, you can explain, feelings are not an excuse for not following directions or doing what is expected of him. You can certainly say, "I understand that you miss your mom. I miss her, too, and we'll discuss that in a few minutes, but it doesn't mean you're not going to bed on time." Likewise, children will say "You don't love me" as a way of diverting a situation. If it's time to make your bed: "You don't love me." If it's time to go to school: "You don't love me." "That's not the issue," you can tell them. "The issue is that you have to make your bed now because we're getting ready to go to school." Of course, always reassure your grandchildren that you love them. Children can't hear "I love you" too much. They just can't use it to get their own way.

• *Try to stay calm.* Sometimes children will push every single button you have, and you won't feel like being nurturing or loving. If you can, stay cool and collected. If you let your grandchildren realize they can get to you, you lose. Once they know they can shake you, it will be an uphill battle to regain control. Also, your grandchildren look to you for security and a sense of order. If you lose your temper, you may just confirm their conviction that all adults, like their parents, are out of control. This doesn't mean that you can't admit fear or sadness or anger, but children need to know that they can trust your stability.

OVERCOMPENSATION

Henrietta Casper has a problem. Her 15-year-old grandson is defiant and disrespectful. When she tells him he can't go out at night, he just walks out the door. Her husband would set firmer rules, but Henrietta can't stick to them. She promised her daughter on her deathbed that she would always care for Adam, and she can't find it in herself even to withhold privileges from the boy. Henrietta is falling into a classic grandparenting trap: overcompensation. She is trying to make up for the pain and the loss her grandchild has suffered by attempting to make him happy every moment, in other words, by always giving him what he wants.

It's an easy trap to fall into. Up until now you have been a grandparent and only a grandparent. You could dote, pamper, spoil, and comfort to your heart's content. It is hard to realize that you are now a surrogate parent and must also discipline and educate your grandchildren. It can take time for this new reality to sink in. Some grandparents can spend years caught between roles; they stay indulgent grandparents, rarely letting a day go by without buying something, however small, for their grandchildren. Then they don't understand why they can't get respect as parents. If you let your grandchildren have French fries and ice cream for breakfast, as one grandma did, it's hard to make them eat vegetables at dinner. You can't spoil them and educate them at the same time; you only send them mixed messages.

Grandparents who overcompensate do so materially and emotionally. Not only do they try to soothe their grandchildren with presents and surprises, but they overlook setting limits. They make allowances they never would have made with their own children. For instance, one day my mother told Kevin that he couldn't watch television until he made his bed. An hour later, I found Kevin in front of the television, and my mother was making his bed. She never would have done that with us.

It is important to realize that overcompensation doesn't help a child in the long run. No matter how much you do for your grandchildren, you cannot remove the pain, repair the loss, or fill the void that is inside them. The world has taken away more than you can put back. Nor do you do your grandchildren any favors by giving in. Children need limits to know they are loved and to develop a sense of who they are. All overcompensating does is teach them to expect permissiveness; it lets them feel that the world owes them things and that they don't have to behave or work to have them. This sense of entitlement can cause all kinds of other problems later in life. Your grandchildren need to deal with their losses in the best way they can, with support and guidance from you and the other adults in their lives. They need a combination of nurturing and discipline, and they need consistency in both. They need to know that you will do what you say you will do, even when they may not like the outcome.

You can't make up for your grandchildren's past, but with time and patience you can build a foundation of trust, love, and security in the present. Real parenting doesn't bring the immediate smiles and laughter that presents do—sometimes it brings sour looks and loud complaints—but remember that you are doing more than making your grandchildren happy in the moment. You are giving these children the necessary tools to grow and build their futures.

PARENTING 101

Beth Grafton had already raised seven children of her own, so she was insulted when the judge who granted her custody of her grandchildren sent her and her husband to parenting classes. He was, she discovered, a prudent man. It had been 30 years since she had raised her own children, and those years, she came to realize, do make a difference. Grandparents who become surrogate parents are often ill equipped for the job. Childrearing has changed since you raised your own children, as has the society in which you raised them.

Children have changed. Through television, the Internet, and other media, this generation knows more about sex, violence, and the world around them and at an earlier age than their parents did. And if your grandchildren came from a drug-using or abusive home, they may know even more about the adult world than other kids their age. The threats of drugs, gangs, and disease, combined with peer pressure, create additional parenting problems you weren't faced with 20 or 30 years ago, as can new challenges caused by rapidly changing technology.

Standards have also changed. Many disciplinary actions you may have used in the past are no longer accepted as parenting techniques. In fact, some are considered abusive. Frances Morgan, like many parents of the old school, used to wash her kids' mouths out with soap when they were small; today that would be grounds for removing a child from her home.

Some grandparents are shy of parenting. They feel they made mistakes with their own children and don't want to repeat them with their grandchildren. Others have been away from childrearing so long that they have forgotten how kids behave. They don't have a clear perspective on what is acceptable behavior and what should be disciplined.

Like Beth Grafton's judge, I recommend that grandparents look into parenting classes. You will find them offered through child guidance clinics, family service agencies, hospitals, and even local colleges. It's not that you are necessarily doing anything wrong with your grandchildren, but parenting classes can teach you new methods for helping them learn responsibility, accountability, confidence, and self-esteem. They can also help you sort through issues that weren't even on the table when you first raised children.

Grandparent support groups are also a good resource. Grandparents who have taken classes are often happy to share their new knowledge with others in the group, and you may hear techniques you haven't tried. Perhaps your group could persuade a child psychologist to hold a parenting seminar specifically for grandparents.

If you don't have access to groups or classes, you can avail yourself of the many good parenting books and websites out there. Moreover, there is a whole world of popular magazines and blogs that regularly run articles and encourage conversations about common childrearing problems and innovative solutions.

What follows is a brief list of the principles and techniques that might be taught today in Parenting 101:

- *Beware of physical punishment.* There is a fine line between discipline and abuse in handling children, a fine line between evoking respect and fear. Today, hitting a child with anything other than a hand on clothing may be construed as child abuse, and you cannot lay a hand on a child who is placed with you through children's services. I don't ever advocate spanking children. When you hit children, you teach them that anger and aggression are acceptable ways to solve problems. You teach fear instead of respect. It is much better for children to learn that actions have consequences. That kind of lesson lays the groundwork for better decision making as they grow older.

- *Reinforce good behavior.* Your grandchildren know that bad behavior will get your attention. And that is often what they want, regardless of how they get it. Therefore, the best way to create good behavior is to *pay attention to it*—with praise and rewards. Try to catch your grandchildren in the act of being good. Be specific in your praise; let them know exactly what behavior you like. Tell them that you see they are making an effort. Behavior charts and chore charts let children keep track of the good things they've done and give them a way to measure their progress toward a reward: an allowance, an ice-cream cone, a special day at the park with Grandpa.

- *Try time-out.* If your grandchild does misbehave, one of the more popular techniques in modern parenting is the use of a time-out. This resembles the old scenario of a child sitting in a corner, but it is meant more as a calming technique than as a punishment. Time-out involves removing a disruptive child from the situation in which he is misbehaving and giving him time to cool off. It doesn't have to be a long time, just long enough to give him time to think about his actions. The actual amount of time will depend on the age of the child—a good rule of thumb is one minute per year of age—but use a timer so that he knows that the length of time is not arbitrary. When the child returns to the situation, make sure he understands which behavior warranted the time-out. Communication is important in any discipline technique.

• *Make your consequences natural, logical, and appropriate.* The goal of discipline is to teach children to regulate themselves, to make them responsible for their actions. Discipline works best when you can link the consequence to the behavior, teaching the child important lessons about cause and effect. If a child throws food on the wall, she must clean it up (even if you have to do it again after she goes to bed). If she insists on wearing shoes that are too small, let her wear them. If they hurt, she won't wear them tomorrow. If your grandson refuses to wear a sweater to school, let him go. If he's a little chilly in class, he'll wear one tomorrow without your nagging. Of course, allowing children to learn from their own mistakes doesn't apply in situations that affect their health and safety or anyone else's.

• *Make consequences immediate.* Children, particularly young ones, have short memories and a poor sense of time. They may not remember why they can't watch television tonight if they are being disciplined for something they did in the morning. Try to make consequences as immediate as possible; it makes them more effective and teaches the concept of cause and effect.

• *Reinforce cause and effect.* Children also have short attention spans. For any consequence or discipline to be effective, the child must connect the cause and the effect. For instance, if you give Susie a time-out for throwing sand in her brother's face, she may need help connecting the two events. Therefore, ask her at the end of the time-out why it was used. If she can say, "Because I threw sand at Tommy instead of using my words," she will not only remember why she was disciplined but will learn responsibility for her actions. The same principle applies with older children when you take away cell phone or computer privileges.

• *Teach responsibility.* Children do many things to test your reactions; they also do things they don't know are wrong. Sometimes it's worth letting one misbehavior go in order to teach responsibility. For instance, if John throws food at the wall, it doesn't hurt to give him another chance, provided he understands that if he does it again, he won't get to finish dinner, he'll have to clean up the mess, or he'll have a time-out. If he throws food at the wall again, he does it knowing what will happen. Again, discipline involves teaching children to regulate themselves; that means letting them make choices and take responsibility for the consequences.

- *Don't make empty threats.* It is never a good idea to threaten children; simply teach them that there are consequences to their behavior. If Joan doesn't do her chores, she can't go online. If Mark hits his brother, he may have to spend time alone in his room without computer or telephone access. But make sure that the consequences are those that you, as the voice of authority, can follow through with. Grandparents have a particularly hard time setting limits and holding to them. You feel bad, you want to be nice, you give in. Thus, you end up teaching the children that they can get whatever they want if they make you feel bad. "No television for a month" is a great threat—but an empty one if you can't keep it. Withhold television privileges for the week, or even the night, and the children will learn that their actions have consequences. (Besides, if you do ban television for a month, you may be punishing yourself as well.)

- *Pick your battles.* Not every misbehavior is cause for confrontation. Some things can be calmly diverted and others simply ignored. If Mary Anne is writing on the table, try giving her paper first. The problem may stop there. Did Todd leave the room cursing under his breath because you forbade texting at the table? Try letting it go. If he is disrespectful to your face, you need to deal with it, but he is entitled to feel unhappy and resentful and to express his feelings to himself. If you make each and every improper action into a crisis, you'll only squander your energy and foster a terrible relationship with your grandchild. Weigh the pros and cons before you make an issue of something. Ask yourself, "What do I expect to gain and what do I want the child to learn from this?" Then pick your battles accordingly.

- *Plan for prevention.* Kids are growing up faster today than ever, it seems, and while teen pregnancy rates have declined in recent years, teen moms still account for nearly half a million babies born in the United States each year.[4] Don't stick your head in the sand. Be proactive, and educate your grandchildren—girls and boys—about birth control, sexually transmitted diseases (STDs), and sexual responsibility. It doesn't mean you condone early sexual activity; it means you are thinking ahead to keep them safe. The reality is that, after a certain age, you can't control what your grandchildren do; you can't be with them every second. But you can give them enough information and tools to make responsible decisions.

PARENTING IN A VIRTUAL WORLD

For nine years, Melinda Squires had had guardianship of her son's three children. Dad had lost custody due to substance abuse issues, and Mom was incarcerated in Texas. When Mom got out of jail, she friended her oldest son, Sammy, online by posing as a teenager. She gained his trust, then disclosed that she was his mother. She secretly sent him a cell phone so they could communicate. One night, she came to San Francisco, and Sammy ran away with her.

Phyllis and Randy Michaels had adopted their two grandsons. Their mother had died of a drug overdose when the boys were small, and their father, Jeff, was simply not interested in parenting. Both boys were on ball teams and friends with their coach's kids. Coach, meanwhile, was friends with Dad. Phyllis had told Coach that she didn't want the boys on Facebook. Jeff was constantly posting things about drinking, partying, girlfriends, and visits to Chicago that did not include his children, and she didn't want them to see it. Unfortunately, Coach disrespected her wishes and let the boys online at his house. It sent them spiraling into horrible behavior and depression.

Technology changes parenting—and grandparenting—in ways we can't ever anticipate. And each wave of change seems to lead to more freedoms for young people, and less control to those who care for them. Computers, cell phones, social networking sites, and texting all give kids a communication stream that is mostly invisible to the adults around them. Meanwhile, technology changes so quickly that whatever you are comfortable with will be, by definition, a generation or two behind your grandkids. It's tempting to give in to intimidation and bury your head in the sand—to hide behind "I'm too old for all this." Don't do it. The virtual world can be every bit as worrisome as the physical world. And while you can't shield your grandchild from this world any more than you can lock him away from strangers and heartbreak, you *can* educate him, supervise him, and equip him with the tools to make good choices.

• *Get with the program.* Whatever technology your grandchild is using, get active and fluent with it. Step into the child's world of communication and talk to her in her own technology. Is she texting? Learn to text. Is he involved with social networking? Join the network. Are they into gaming? Learn enough about gaming to talk to them, to understand what they're engaged with.

- *Take the second chair.* Talk to your grandkids about what you're doing and what they're doing. Dr. Gigi Johnson, a media expert, calls it "the second chair phenomenon."[5] Pull up a chair and show them what you're doing on the computer, just as you would show them in the kitchen or garden. Pull up a chair and ask about what they're doing. Encourage them to teach you, if they know more. Letting them be your teacher can build their confidence and create a great bonding experience. This is different from looking over their shoulder, though. Kids have a whole list of codes that lets their friends know when an adult is hovering over their shoulder.

- *Start early.* It's never too early to educate your grandchildren about safety. You probably already have systems in place for talking to them about crossing the street, good neighborhoods, bad neighborhoods, and not talking to strangers. This is really an extension of that conversation. Technology has created a virtual community composed of good and bad neighborhoods, populated by wonderful educators and entertainers as well as invisible strangers and cyberbullies. Your grandchildren will be communicating with a lot of people you don't know. Be active, concerned, and interested, and make your grandchildren aware of the risks.

- *Set clear expectations.* Just as you set expectations and boundaries around bedtime, curfews, and public behavior, you can set expectations about technology use: That you will be one of their friends online. That they will answer if you call their cell phone. That texting you does not imply permission; they must wait for you to respond. That all this costs money, and they must respect your family's budgetary restraints. That certain times and locations are off limits for phone calls, texting, and computer use. That what happens on the computer is not private, since you're legally responsible for what they do online. Communicate as clearly, openly, and *nondefensively* on this topic as you would in any other area of family expectations. After all, technology can also be your friend. "Kids today are often willing to text you where they are with much more frequency than you would have told your parents," says Dr. Johnson.[6] "A negotiated text when they change locations can provide both sides with peace of mind."

- *Make media a family affair.* Invite connected media into the living room TV, if you can. You can stream old movies and play games through various Internet sites, while devices like the Wii and Xbox Kinect can have the whole family bowling and dancing together. You might also want to think about laptops and tablets instead of desktop computers. This way the kids can be on their computers doing homework or connecting with friends but still be in your company, where you can keep an eye on them.

• *Protect yourself.* Children are not the only ones at risk online. Some sites that offer cartoons, free games, animé, and other things that appeal to kids may also hide viruses, worms, information thieves, and other predators that put you and your computer in danger. Not only do you need to educate your grandkids, you need to protect your private information. Make sure you install current security programs and regularly clear your hard drive.

• *Track behavior, when you can.* Just as you may check outside trash cans when you've been out for a while (and if you don't, you should, as kids don't often think to remove telltale signs of misbehavior from the property), you should periodically check the history folders on their computers. It will tell you where they've been wandering online. There are also many digital tracking tools, offered by many reputable companies, which will run in the background and let you passively watch for trends. Don't take these as absolutes, however. Dr. Johnson's own kids realized that they could reset one of these tools if they just got their own copy and reinstalled it.[7]

• *Educate yourself.* Learn about tracking programs, blocking programs, and Internet and cell phone safety. Look online for community programs, books, and websites that help parents address these issues. Of course, kids are good at hacking safety programs, but that doesn't mean you should give up on them.

• *Be photo conscious.* Everything is so fast these days. You take a picture at a birthday party, and in the time it takes to blow out the candles, the image is already online. Schools often have online websites with snapshots of events. It is worth thinking about who takes pictures of your grandchildren and where they end up, especially if you are trying to limit a disruptive parent's access to them. Even nuclear families are careful about having children's photos or names online these days. Consider your situation and your stance on public photos. If you are concerned about keeping pictures off the Web, talk to the school, scouting groups, and other parents; let them know.

• *Talk to other parents.* "Our parents used to ask questions when we'd go visit people: Is there a gun in the house? Is there a pool? Is there a parent home?" says Johnson. "No one ever asks, 'What kind of computer access will my children have? What kinds of games do you run? What will the kids do while they're there?'" If, like Phyllis Michaels, you want to limit your grandchildren's exposure to certain sites, speak clearly with their friends' parents. You can't control whether or not they respect your wishes, but you can control whether your grandkids go there again if they don't.

THE HYPERACTIVE GRANDCHILD

Jewell Baxter's grandsons are three and four years old, and they are out of control. They have put silverware down the toilet and painted the walls with toothpaste. They urinated in the furnace and flooded the kitchen floor when Grandpa fell asleep (the floor alone cost Jewell $750 to fix). "You can't leave them alone a second," she says. "You just can't fall asleep!" If Emily Petersen turns around for a second, four-year-old Amanda is down under the house or up in the attic. Emily isn't physically able to crawl around looking for her when she disappears and is terrified that the little girl will get seriously hurt. Six-year-old Gregory can barely control himself in school. He is a smart child, but he cannot sit still long enough to complete his assignments. Now he has begun to kick and beat up other children. Even in GAP meetings he bounces off walls. "I'm going to hang that little boy!" says his grandmother in frustration.

Sound familiar? Then you could very well have a hyperactive child on your hands.

A large percentage of the grandchildren I see and hear about are hyperactive, part of a condition called *attention-deficit/hyperactivity disorder,* or ADHD[8] (it's often referred to as *attention deficit disorder,* or ADD, when there is no hyperactivity involved). ADHD affects up to nine percent of school-age children, or approximately 1 in 10 kids.[9] The U.S. Surgeon General calls it "the most commonly diagnosed behavioral disorder of childhood."[10] ADHD is believed to be a neurological condition caused by heredity, medical problems, or prenatal exposure to drugs and alcohol. The result is difficulty with attention, concentration, impulsiveness, and self-control.

Simply put, children with ADHD have trouble concentrating, completing a task, sitting still, and focusing. They are easily distracted, are disruptive, and may have poor relationships with other children. They have little impulse control, acting before they think about the consequences of their behavior. They may get themselves into dangerous situations and not know why or how they happened. They require constant supervision, which can be exhausting for grandparents who may not have the energy or patience they once had.

Children with ADHD may be bright and yet do poorly in school, which can lead to their believing they are failures or bad kids. Poor self-image and low self-esteem are deep issues with these children. They don't mean to drive you crazy; their bodies just seem to move faster than their brains. One little girl came crying to her grandmother after acting up in school one day. "I don't know why I did those things," she said. "I don't know what happens to me, because I didn't want to do them."

Of course, not every child who gets into trouble in school or has difficulty concentrating is hyperactive. Some children appear to be hyperactive when the problem is really a learning disability or an emotional disturbance. A lot of kids who get labeled with ADHD are suffering from grief, loss, and trauma. And sometimes a child can experience a combination of the three. On the other hand, many children with ADHD are not hyperactive but may still exhibit difficulties with attention and/or impulsive behavior (they may be referred to as having ADD). As with any disability, the various symptoms of ADHD and ADD may range from mild to severe, depending on the individual child and even the specific situation (some children may exhibit more problems in school or social settings than at home).

If you suspect your grandchild has ADHD or ADD, have him or her evaluated by a well-trained professional—a child psychologist, child psychiatrist, or a pediatrician who has training and experience in this area. There is no simple test for ADHD; a true diagnosis is pieced together, like a puzzle, from a variety of elements, including family and medical histories, a physical exam, psychological testing, screening for learning disabilities, and interviews with the child's caregivers and teachers. You can start the evaluation process through the school or community mental health clinic; some states provide early intervention services for children as young as one or two years old (see Chapter 13). You can also have your grandchild assessed by a private doctor. Mental health clinics and parent or grandparent support groups are good sources of referrals. If your grandchild is positively diagnosed with ADHD (or ADD), he or she should be referred to a child psychiatrist or psychologist for treatment, which should include counseling and may involve medication.

Medication for ADHD

ADHD is a complex disorder, and there are some disagreements about how to treat it. Perhaps one of the main issues under debate is the use of prescription drugs. Stimulant drugs, like Ritalin, seem to have a calming effect on children with ADHD and are the most common type of medication used to manage it, although nonstimulant medications and some antidepressants have also been used in treatment.

Proponents of medication applaud its effectiveness in reducing restlessness and impulsive behavior and thus helping a child concentrate and focus. Properly prescribed, such drugs have allowed a calmer existence for hyperactive children, their families, friends, and teachers and have enabled these children to improve their school and social performance and feel better about themselves.

Critics, however, feel that doctors may be overmedicating children and are concerned about side effects, which can range from moodiness and insomnia to abnormally rapid heartbeats, nervousness, and lack of appetite. Meanwhile, parents—and grandparents—of children with ADHD must work with their doctors to make informed decisions based on the individual child and his or her particular needs.

I was not originally an advocate of medicating children, but I have seen hyperactive kids do a complete turnaround with the right prescription and dosage. In fact, many people compare the effects of the right medication to putting glasses on a nearsighted person; glasses don't change the physical makeup of the eye, but they do let everything come into focus. Like glasses, these drugs can be a tool, not a solution. However, finding the right medication and the proper dosage may take trial and error and patience. Nor does every child respond well to medication.

Talk to your grandchild's doctor carefully. Ask lots of questions. Consider all your options. Above all, if you do decide to use medication, make sure your grandchild is closely monitored by doctors on a regular basis. Look for any changes or reactions to the drugs. Try to involve teachers in the monitoring process as well; they will notice changes in school that you might not see at home. Make sure the treatment program is a well-rounded one. Medication alone will not cause long-term changes. Nor will it cure depression or anxiety. Your grandchild also needs a combina-

Could Your Grandchild Have ADHD?

If a number of the following symptoms describe your grandchild, particularly if they started before age seven, and if they have lasted at least six months, you may have reason to suspect ADHD or ADD. However, a definite diagnosis requires a full examination by a qualified doctor.[11]

- Has difficulty concentrating
- Shifts excessively from one activity to another
- Often does not seem to listen
- Has difficulty following instructions
- Often fails to finish things he or she starts
- Has difficulty organizing
- Often loses things
- Is easily distracted
- Is frequently forgetful
- Fidgets or squirms excessively
- Has difficulty staying seated
- Has difficulty playing quietly
- Often blurts out answers to questions
- Often acts before thinking
- Often talks excessively
- Has difficulty waiting
- Often engages in dangerous activities

tion of therapy and behavior modification to internalize and learn to use new behaviors.

WHEN YOUR GRANDCHILD NEEDS THERAPY

My own feeling is that most children who are taken in by grandparents could use some kind of counseling to handle the adjustment. Most could benefit from therapy, even as a preventive measure. Groups are great because each child realizes that he or she is not the only one with disturbing feelings. Most of these kids have such terrible self-esteem that even short-term therapy can help them understand that none of this is their fault. Children who act out their frustrations will often come to the attention of the school, which may then refer them to counseling. Unfortunately, the children who don't act out—the quiet ones or the good students—may slip through the cracks.

Does your grandchild need therapy? Counseling is especially important if any of the following statements describe your grandchild:

- The child has been physically or sexually abused.
- The child begins to remember past abuse. Sometimes you know the child was abused; sometimes this information only becomes available when something triggers the memories and a flood of painful emotions is released.
- The child seems depressed, particularly if he or she has been abused. (Remember, even very young children get depressed; observe your grandchild closely.)
- The child has been exhibiting behavioral, psychological, emotional, medical, or academic problems for a noticeable or prolonged period of time.
- The child is experiencing extreme fear or extreme anger.
- The child is sexually acting out.
- The child is constantly fighting or exhibits cruel behavior. (Often, kids who have been abused will then abuse their siblings, peers, and pets.)
- The child exhibits a combination of bed-wetting, fire setting, and cruelty to animals.

- The child becomes self-destructive, talks about hurting himself, or shows hints of wanting to die. People think young children don't think about wanting to die, but they do. The danger signs include any potentially self-destructive behavior, from walking out in front of cars to expressing thoughts of feeling unloved or saying, "I wish I weren't here." A child who lives with you because of a death may talk about wanting to be with Mom or Dad in heaven. Behavior like this is always a cry for help. Even if your grandchild uses it as a tool to manipulate you—and if he knows it gets to you, he could use it that way—it still masks deeper issues and needs to be dealt with in counseling.

RESIDENTIAL PLACEMENT

Seven-year-old Matthew had witnessed the murder of his father by his mother and was becoming dangerously aggressive in school and at home; on one occasion he tried to smother his younger sister. Nine-year-old Jesse had been physically and sexually abused before he came to live with his grandparents; he later started to act out sexually with his younger siblings. Sally, 10, is rebellious. She refuses to listen to her grandmother and repeatedly disappears from school and home. One night she cut the window screen and slipped out of the house with her grandmother's car keys, which she gave to a stranger who then stole the car; she didn't reappear until 1:00 A.M. and would not say where she had been. Six-year-old Nicholas is destructive. He tears plaster off walls and throws things at his grandmother. He was born with drugs in his system and is severely hyperactive. He, too, will often sneak out of the house at night for hours.

Unfortunately, some children need more help than a grandparent can give them. They lack the ability to express their pain in words, and their actions put them and others in jeopardy. Some, like Matthew and Jesse, have experienced such deep trauma that they cannot control their behavior. Others, like Nicholas, are driven by chemical and neurological problems. Medication for hyperactivity, weekly outpatient therapy, and a grandma's love are not enough for these children. They need the more intense therapy that a residential program can offer.

A residential program is a live-in facility where children can receive round-the-clock professional care. A social worker or school psychologist often makes the recommendation to place a child in residential treatment, but grandparents can also request placement through the proper channels. Sally's grandmother, for instance, called child protective services and told them that her granddaughter was placing herself in danger and that she, as an ailing 80-year-old, could no longer handle her. Matthew, on the other hand, was placed through the department of mental health after a school evaluation found him to be severely emotionally disturbed.

Children who are placed through child protective services become dependents of the court, and their grandparents lose control over what happens to them. This is not so for children, like Matthew, who enter residential facilities through other channels; their grandparents may retain some control over their welfare even while they are in placement.

Giving up your grandchild to a treatment center is not an easy decision to make. It practically tore Nicholas's grandmother apart. "I look at Nicholas sleeping, and I cry," she admits. "But he is getting bad. Nicholas cannot help himself, and I don't have the knowledge to help him help himself." Nor is placement always a grandparent's decision. Sometimes grandparents don't recognize that they can't provide the home or guidance a severely disturbed child needs; in these cases the social worker may recommend placement over the grandparent's objections.

Placement, for any child, is an absolute last resort. No grandparent wants to put a grandchild in a facility, but if you have done everything in your power to help a child, and if she needs more than you can provide or is a danger to herself and others, residential placement may be your only option. It doesn't mean that you don't love your grandchild or that you are abandoning her. You can still maintain contact through letters, phone calls, and visits. What it does mean is that you are giving the child her best chance to become a healthy, happy, productive adult.

GRATITUDE VERSUS GROWTH

Children are very self-centered; they have a tough time looking outside themselves. This is particularly true of children who have suffered loss. You may want them to be grateful for your hard work and sacrifices, but it is unreasonable to expect gratitude from a child who has been traumatized and who is angry about the situation. As adults they might look back and appreciate what you did for them, but right now they are just getting by.

It's ironic that the better the job you do parenting your grandchildren, the more likely you are to be taken for granted. Don't let it upset you. It means that your grandchildren have come to expect your love and attention and that it is not a rare treat in their lives. Take heart, instead, at the good you are doing.

Many children thrive under their grandparent's care—even those who were abandoned and abused. In a study that interviewed kids being raised by grandparents, and even great-grandparents, the children reported feeling "safe, cared for and loved." Yes, they felt rejection and disappointment with their parents, and yes, they had histories that included abuse and neglect, but they also had friends, expressed themselves artistically, were achieving in school and sports, and were optimistic about the future.[12]

It is a testament to the quality of the grandparent–grandchild relationship. "These kids are at high risk for emotional problems," a psychologist once told the *Orange County Register.* "The fact that they aren't suffering those problems shows how resilient kids are. And what a good job a lot of grandparents are doing raising grandchildren."[13]

7

Your Grandchild
and the School

The hardest thing about school was adjusting with my friends.
I really didn't understand my situation—how could they
understand it?

—*Kevin, age 19*

Jeffrey Campos, age six, has a hard time settling down to his studies.
Alternately shutting down and acting out, easily stimulated and hyperactive, he can't function well in large classrooms. "Grandma, I can't
stand the noise," he confesses when he comes home. "There's too much
noise—people talking all the time!" The teachers say Jeffrey is intelligent,
but he gets frustrated and overwhelmed. "For a while he didn't want to
go to school at all," says his grandmother. "He thought he was stupid and
couldn't do what the other kids were doing."

Heather Pierce, 10, has trouble reading; although she is in the fourth
grade, she reads at a second-grade level. She loves books but feels "dumb
and stupid" because other children do so much better than she does. For
their part, the other kids make fun of Heather.

Schoolwork is not a problem for five-year-old Bobby Franklin, but the
classroom is. That is where he takes out most of his frustration, by acting
out and fighting with other children. Generally, Bobby is an average kid

in terms of behavior—sometimes he listens, sometimes he doesn't—but after he has had a visit with his mother, he becomes a minor terror in school.

School is rough for many kids. They get hassled about what they wear, they're expected to act a certain way, and they feel foolish if they're too different. And that's just with the other children. Strict teachers, rules and regulations, and the challenge of schoolwork itself can add new levels of stress to a child's life. But for a child being raised by grandparents, especially for a child with emotional or academic difficulties, school can be a minefield of problems, from social isolation to failing a grade.

BEING DIFFERENT: ODD CHILD OUT

Most children want to fit in, whether it is to the group playing hopscotch on the sidewalk or to the class on a school picnic. Children raised by grandparents suffer the stigma of being raised in a family that is different. And other children can be cruel about differences. Not only do they seem to have radar to seek them out, but their playground teasing can be merciless. Fourteen-year-old Tyler remembers attending a parochial school in Boston where everyone knew that he lived with his grandmother, that his mother was an addict, and that his father was dead. The teasing was mean. The other kids cursed his mother and called her foul names; they said that his father killed himself because of Tyler and that his mom took off because he was ugly. Tyler admits, "The part that got me was they said my mom left me because she didn't really want me."

Adults face peer pressure in the workplace; children find it in the school yard. Even innocent childhood jokes can take on different, and painful, meanings for children who are surviving a loss. "I'm a little more sensitive to certain things than most of my friends," says my nephew Kevin. "When I got to middle school, people would rag on each other, just with friends. It was nothing serious, but they would start telling momma jokes, and stuff like that. I would take it personally, even though I knew they were joking around." The same kind of jokes started at least one fight in high school. "I don't remember what the kid said," Kevin admits. "It didn't matter what he had said . . . just that he had said it."

Not only do your grandchild's peers make insensitive comments about the fact that you are older than their parents, but most school activities presume a parent–child relationship: from making Mother's and Father's Day cards to parent–teacher conferences. This can be troubling for the child who doesn't have a mother or doesn't know where she is.

BEHAVIOR PROBLEMS IN SCHOOL

All the emotional and behavioral problems your grandchildren experience at home may be exacerbated when they start school, and new ones may become apparent. Anxiety, fear of abandonment, and clingy behavior may take on new dimensions in a school setting. Your grandchildren face hours of not knowing where you are, how you are, and if you are coming back. Just taking them to school can be a trial if they are afraid you won't pick them up again. Some children even develop phantom health problems so you'll come and take them home.

Nor are school personnel always understanding. Ten-year-old Kirsten was tense and anxious after her grandmother had bypass surgery. Every time she heard an ambulance pass the school, she panicked. All day she asked if she could call home, just to make sure her grandma was fine, but the teachers refused her requests, believing that Kirsten was using the situation to manipulate them.

Anger, aggression, and inappropriate behavior may also find new outlets, and new triggers, in school. A little boy who has trouble with authority may defy his teachers. A little girl who is verbally or physically aggressive at home may hit or swear at other children. Your grandchildren may be bossy and have trouble making and keeping friends, which may only make them angrier. Many grandchildren only know how to get negative attention. They know how to push the buttons of their teachers and peers, just as they know how to push yours. They may get labeled as problem children or acquire a reputation as poor students. They may skip school. Some may even fail and have to repeat grades.

On the other hand, withdrawn, depressed children may become introspective and shy at school. They seem to disappear in class. Their attitude is this: "If I sit in the back of the room and don't open my mouth, I won't get in trouble because they won't know I'm here." These children often get lost in the cracks. Loner kids may be viewed by teachers as a relief, as one less problem child to deal with. They may get good grades, but they may also slip by with C's and D's because they don't cause trouble; unfortunately, they may not learn anything, either.

New behavior problems in grandchildren may also appear in a classroom setting: difficulty following directions, difficulty playing with other children, difficulty waiting their turn. Many of the characteristics of attention-deficit/hyperactivity disorder (ADHD) and learning disabilities only come to the surface once a child starts school.

ADHD IN THE CLASSROOM AND SCHOOL YARD

As I mentioned in Chapter 6, many of the grandchildren I see and hear about have ADHD, which means they have trouble with attention and concentration; may be easily distracted, restless, or hyperactive; and are given to impulsive behavior. Although all children are inattentive, impulsive, and overly active from time to time, children with ADHD seem to be that way most of the time. For them such behavior is the rule, not the exception.

Children with ADHD face many challenges in school. They may have a hard time adapting to the classroom setting, performing their schoolwork, and acquiring the social skills necessary to make friends and play in groups. Children who have trouble with attention may have a hard time following directions or finishing projects. Long reading assignments and tests may be particularly difficult. If they are not hyperactive, they may be inattentive and underactive, appearing to daydream or wander off. They may be labeled "lazy" or "spacey" and accused of not trying. If they are hyperactive, they may be disruptive in class, constantly moving and unable to stay in their seats. Like Jeffrey Campos, they may be easily overstimulated and overwhelmed by a large, noisy classroom. If they are impulsive, they will act without thinking, calling out in class or blurting out answers before the questions are asked.

These traits may carry over to the playground, where children typically hone their social skills. A child with ADHD may interrupt other children's games or make jokes at the wrong moment. He may not be able to wait his turn, or he may frustrate easily and overreact. His behavior can lead to difficulty making friends, which can lower his self-esteem.

Each child with ADHD will demonstrate different symptoms and in different intensities, but the result will be a disorganized approach to learning and developing and a difficult time keeping pace with children his age. These children are not stupid. In fact, you may hear this remark from teachers: "Your grandchild! He is smart enough to do the work, if he would only *try*." It is not a question of intelligence but of attention and self-control. An informed teacher may recognize these behaviors as symptoms of ADHD. Unfortunately, an uninformed teacher may blame the child.

LEARNING DISABILITIES: THE INTERNAL STUMBLING BLOCKS

April Thomas was miserable in grade school. Reading assignments took forever, classes seemed to rush by too fast, and tests were a nightmare. She would look at words on the blackboard and not realize she was reading them backward. She would struggle with a book and come away with only bits and pieces of the story. She would listen to her teacher's instructions but not exactly understand what was required of her. Some teachers got impatient with her many questions, so she stopped asking. "I would sit in class and pretend I understood what the teacher was saying," April, now 20, recalls. "Most of the time I didn't, but I was too embarrassed to admit it."

Because she was a bright girl, April was accused of "playing dumb" and of not trying hard enough. She was actually trying very hard, but it was a struggle to understand the questions, let alone come up with answers. Eventually, April got frustrated and gave up. She didn't want to seem stupid, so she became rebellious, making wisecracks in class. And she fell further and further behind her peers.

In high school April was finally diagnosed with learning disabilities. She received a tutor, special classes, extended time to take tests and turn in papers, and other modifications. Today she is a sophomore in college. April has learned to compensate for her learning problems and to enlist the help of teachers and administrators when she needs more time for assignments or permission to tape a lecture. Still, she is shy about her disability. "It's extra embarrassing because it is an invisible disability," she says. "If I had one leg shorter than the other and couldn't run fast, it would be a reason that people could see."

People may not be able to see April's disabilities, but many other children would understand them. Approximately one out of every five people in the United States is affected by a learning disability, and about five percent of all school-age children receive special education services to help them compensate for different problems.[1]

Children who have learning disabilities may experience problems with reading comprehension, spoken language, writing and spelling, arithmetic, reasoning, and organizational skills. They may also exhibit symptoms of ADHD. In fact, many learning-disabled kids also have ADHD. Like children with ADHD, learning-disabled children are not dumb. They do not lack intelligence or a desire to learn. They have a problem with how they interpret outside information, a deficit in the psychological mechanisms that process selective visual, auditory, or tactile data. Learning disabilities must not be confused with problems due to mental retardation, serious emotional disturbance, or sensory deficits like blindness or deafness, which fall into other categories of disabilities.

Just because your grandchild has trouble with math or spelling, however, does not mean she has a learning disability. Many people experience learning *difficulties*—certain subjects they don't take to easily; there are, for example, children who love reading but hate science or who just don't seem to have a head for numbers. However, if your grandchild's problems are so constant or severe that they disrupt her education or day-to-day activities (such as reading street signs or using the telephone) or if there is a significant gap between the child's academic potential and academic achievement that is not the result of environmental, cultural, or economic disadvantage, then you may suspect a learning disability.

MISSED SCHOOL DAYS AND OTHER EDUCATIONAL HAZARDS

Not every child who has problems in school has ADHD or a learning disability. Your grandson may be behind in school simply because he missed too many school days before he came to live with you. Perhaps he was constantly on the move and changing schools with his parents. Perhaps drugs were involved, and getting a child ready for school wasn't the parent's priority. Your grandchild could arrive at a new school a grade or two behind, unable to read, and convinced he is stupid. He may also resist your insistence on regular school attendance, since he never had to attend school regularly before. Here, again, routine and consistency may start to correct the problem.

Another reason a child may do badly is worry. Your granddaughter may display a lack of attention in class because she is thinking about her parents and her circumstances. It can be difficult to complete class assignments, even to listen to the teacher, when a child feels the weight of the world on her shoulders.

Of course, difficulty with schoolwork could also be an indicator of a medical problem. Maybe Tommy does badly in school because he can't see the blackboard or has trouble hearing the teacher. Glasses or a hearing aid could be the answer.

■ HOW TO COPE

• *Talk to the teachers.* Whether your grandchild is hyperactive, acting out, or grieving, I recommend creating open lines of communication with the school. Talk to the teachers, counselors, and the principal; give them insight into your situation. Let them know that if your granddaughter misbehaves when she comes to class on Monday, there may be a reason. Explain that if she had a visit with a parent on the weekend, she is probably reeling with emotions, not simply being obnoxious. Often teachers are more understanding if they know there is an explanation behind a child's problem behavior.

If his teacher understands that Johnny lives with his grandparents and doesn't know where his mother is, she might be more sensitive to his reaction to making a Mother's Day card in class. Maybe she'll have the children make cards for "someone who is special" instead, since not all children live with their mothers or fathers. Having a teacher recognize such a circumstance may give it legitimacy in a child's eyes, and that recognition may soften the stigma of not having a parent to make a card for. The nuclear family of a mom, a dad, and their child is something we can no longer take for granted. Sensitive teachers, being aware of this, have learned to reference grandparents, aunts, uncles, foster parents, and adoptive parents in their lessons or comments about family, family events, and family history.

Your grandchild's teacher may also be your ally in identifying symptoms of ADHD or a learning disability, since some traits may only appear once a child is in school. If you suspect that your grandchild has a developmental or learning problem, share your concerns with the teachers and start to compare notes. If your grandchild does have ADHD or a learning disability, ask what you can do at home to help the child progress.

Of course, many teachers are overwhelmed. They may have 40 kids in a small classroom, each with different problems, and might not be able to give out special help or consideration. Still, the more you can communicate with the teacher, principal, or school counselor, the more your grandchildren will learn about problem solving. If they are children of substance abusers, they have already learned a lot about running away from problems; this is a chance for them to learn that problems can also be worked out. I have on occasion recommended moving a child to a different classroom, but only as a last resort and never before exhausting all other possibilities.

• *Talk to the child.* Jeffrey's grandmother tries to reassure him before tests. "You know it," she tells him. "Just listen and think about what the teacher is asking you, and you're going to be fine. Just do the best you can; we can't ask for more than that." Heather's grandmother tries to keep her from comparing herself to other children. Your own attitudes about learning and the way you communicate them to your grandchildren can influence the way they approach the school experience.

Talk to your grandchildren. Help them emphasize and develop their strengths. Maybe your grandson has trouble with math but is good at basketball, singing, or drawing. Praise him for what he does well, and create opportunities for him to succeed. Every success will boost his self-esteem and encourage him to strive for more success. And teach him to understand his weaknesses. You can reassure him that everyone has some kind of difficulty and that there is no shame in asking for help. Remind him that everyone learns at a different pace and that having difficulty in a subject doesn't mean that he is stupid or dumb or bad. At the same time, don't be so easy on him that you give him permission to give up. His situation may create particular challenges for him in school, but it is not an excuse for him to stop trying. Tell him that he may have to work harder but that he can succeed. Encourage him to keep doing his best. Still, keep your own expectations realistic. If your grandson really does his best, you cannot ask for more.

• *Look into special education.* Just because some children are currently trailing behind the rest of the class does not mean they are doomed to stay behind. Free special education and related services are available to children who are somehow handicapped in the learning process. If there is a chronic problem that prevents your grandchild's schoolwork from matching her intellectual ability, whether it is a learning disability, severe emotional turmoil, or a physical handicap, the child should be eligible for special help through the school system. In fact, most states offer special services to disabled or potentially disabled children before they even enter the school system (see "Start Early," below).

The process of applying for special education will help you and your grandchild uncover the source of her academic troubles and, hopefully, lead to solutions. Sometimes the solution is as simple as obtaining a hearing aid, therapy, or a tutor. It was discovered through testing that one little girl who was doing poorly in school was actually gifted; her poor grades were due to boredom and a lack of confidence.

If your grandchild is having consistent problems in school, try to address them as soon as possible. At least start documenting what you see, and if the situation continues to worsen, request an individualized education program, or IEP (see Chapter 13).

• *Start early.* It is never too early to consider your grandchild's development and learning potential. Children who experience educational and developmental difficulties are often overlooked until they fall severely behind their classmates. By that time, their academic performance has already suffered and they may feel depressed, anxious, and inadequate about school.

You do not have to wait until your grandchild starts school to get the benefits of special education. Physical therapy, speech and language remediation, and other services are often available to children before they even enter kindergarten. Most states offer early intervention programs that are designed to address developmental problems in the preschool years, when children are typically most ready to learn—and at an incredible pace. These preventive programs assume that the earlier children get help, the more chance they have of succeeding later.

If you notice in your grandchild the absence of anything typical for a particular stage of a child's development or any delay in motor coordination, speech, or self-help skills like self-feeding—or if drug exposure or family history have you concerned that problems could develop—look into an early intervention program. Some states even provide services to infants and toddlers. (For more on early intervention, see Chapter 13.)

• *Seek out peer activities.* There is more to a child's school years than simply sitting in a classroom. Extracurricular and recreational experiences are as important for developing social skills as a good education is for developing learning skills. Your grandchild may have taken on many caregiving responsibilities at an early age and may not know how to be just a kid. Scouting organizations, after-school clubs, summer camps, day camps, and athletics provide opportunities for children to *play* with other children and learn to socialize, share, and take turns. Extracurricular activities involving sports, arts, and music also offer children who have academic problems a chance to discover other strengths and build a sense of self-esteem.

• *Find young role models.* Children, particularly those who don't have parents as role models, desperately need the influence of young adults. A younger person may have more energy and stamina than you do. He or she may also understand more clearly the choices and challenges a child faces growing up today, while your ideas may seem old-fashioned. Think about it: just 10 or 15 years (basically anything past their short memories) are an enormity to a child, and two generations is practically ancient. My nephew Kevin used to point out that my parents were "brought up in the old days, like in the time of World War II" (which seemed prehistoric to him). Even kids who have youthful, active grandparents will feel the generational split and may benefit from the influence of younger adults.

Extended family can be a wonderful source of role models for a grandchild, and many grandparents successfully involve aunts and uncles in their grandchildren's lives. In my family, for example, my brother was the one who would play ball with Kevin and take him to sporting events. Beth Grafton's son and daughter-in-law take her grandchildren on vacations. However, not every grandchild has extended family members available. Some aunts and uncles may be caught up with their own families or may live far away, or they may disapprove of your raising the child and therefore keep their distance. Even if the parents were only children, you can still find young adults to interact with your grandchildren. Scouting programs, summer camps, and youth groups bring together children and active young adults, as well as provide fun activities and new experiences for kids. Big Brother and Big Sister programs, and programs like them, exist throughout the country to provide positive role models for children who need them. They can foster caring relationships with lasting connections. I know one little girl whose Big Sister continues to visit her even in a residential facility, and another Big Sister ended up stepping in to assume legal guardianship of a child after her grandma died.

   • *Aim high!* Don't let academic delays or learning disabilities stifle your hopes for your grandchildren. History is full of disabled people who succeeded in the face of tremendous challenges, and many people with learning disabilities have gone on to become scientists, lawyers, generals, even president. Consider the following examples:

> Albert Einstein didn't talk until he was four or read until he was nine; he couldn't learn math through traditional teaching methods. His first teachers thought he was backward. Yet he grew up to win the Nobel Prize in physics and to revolutionize the way we think about space and time.

> Young George Patton couldn't read or write by age 12. Still, he overcame his disabilities and was eventually appointed to the U.S. Military Academy at West Point. He went on to become a general and led the Third Army in Europe during World War II.

> Woodrow Wilson had learning problems as a boy. He was 8 years old before he learned his letters and 11 by the time he learned to read. His relatives considered him "dull and backwards." The only school subject he excelled in was speech. Yet he grew up to become the 28th president of the United States.[2]

   • Is your grandchild a future Einstein, Patton, or Woodrow Wilson? No one can really say. One of the wonders with children is that we don't know what they may become. So help them aim high. The possibilities are all ahead of them.

8

The Drug Epidemic at Home

> Our young people—the young parents—are dead because so
> many of them are hooked on crack. The grandparents are trying
> to save the little ones before the same thing happens to them.
> —*Marin County social worker*[1]

Jim and Fay Strassburger had watched an entire middle-class neighborhood lose child after child to drugs. They could stand in their yard and point to the houses. In one week alone, they attended three funerals for neighbor kids who died of drug-related causes, bright kids who knew the consequences of their actions. Their own son and daughter were still struggling with drug and alcohol addiction; two grandchildren lived with Jim and Fay. "We've lost a whole generation," Jim told a reporter. "Maybe part of the next."[2]

Katherine Connor is raising five drug-exposed grandchildren, all from the same daughter. She can frequently be seen doing her errands with the infant tucked under her arm and the rest of the children trailing after her like a line of small ducks. The mother is on the streets and often violent. She once threw a brick through the kitchen window, almost hitting her own son with a piece of broken glass. When she was picked up by the police, she broke the windows and the grill of the police car—that's how much violent strength she had from her high.

There is no question that we are in the midst of an ongoing drug epidemic. The news is full of stories about local gangs, drug lords, and the victims of drug-related crime. The misuse of prescription medications has exploded into a problem reminiscent of the crack epidemic of the 1980s. Drug-induced deaths have begun to outnumber traffic fatalities in the United States,[3] and overdoses involving painkillers now kill more Americans than cocaine and heroin combined.[4]

But there are other victims: infants exposed to drugs before birth, young children abused and neglected by drug-abusing parents, and grandparents who turn their lives upside down to keep their families together. In the war against drugs, the front line is often at home.

This chapter looks at some of the things you need to know in your own private war on drugs: the truth about addicts and addiction; the symptoms, risks, and needs of drug-exposed children; and suggestions for stopping the cycle of addiction in your grandchildren. Appendix A includes a list of organizations that can provide more detailed information and guidance. Remember, this is a difficult fight, and addiction is a fierce enemy; you can only take each day, and each battle, as it comes.

ABOUT THE ADDICT

There is no way to count how many addicts there really are in this country. According to government statistics, more than 22 million Americans use recreational drugs of some kind (both illegal and prescriptions).[5] And those numbers don't include all prescription drug abusers, those who misuse over-the-counter (OTC) drugs, or kids who start experimenting before the age of 12. The truth is that, for a family struggling with the effects of addiction, even one addict is one too many.

I know grandparents who have spent thousands of dollars and all their energy trying to get their adult children into rehabilitation programs only to see them relapse and return to the streets. They witness the thoughtless abuse and neglect of their grandchildren and are often helpless to protect them. They spend sleepless nights asking the questions: "Where is my child?" "When will he recover?" "Doesn't she see what she's doing to us, to her children, to herself?" "How can we help him?" "Where did we go wrong?" If your adult child is an addict, these questions are probably not strangers to you. But before you can really answer them, you must first understand what addiction is and what it does to the addict.

What Addiction Is

Chemical dependency is not a moral weakness, bad habit, mental illness, or sign of a weak character. It is not a result of life's pressures or a temporary loss of control. Addiction is a disease characterized by a mental and physical dependence on a chemical substance. A person becomes chemically dependent, or addicted, when he or she develops a craving for a substance as a shortcut to feeling pleasure or avoiding pain, including the pain or discomfort of not using the substance itself.

Like many diseases, addiction is chronic, that is, it is constant and long-lasting. Addiction is also progressive in that it gets worse and worse over time, requiring more and more of the substance to achieve the good feelings and prevent the bad ones. And, for some addicts, it can be fatal.

High hopes, good intentions, and promises will not cure the disease of addiction. Intense rehabilitation, strong support, and—for some addicts—medical attention are necessary to bring an addiction under control. Few addictions are truly "cured."

What Addiction Does

Addiction takes over the addict's priorities and makes his behavior unpredictable. The high that originally seduced him gets harder and harder to achieve. It becomes the most important thing in his life—more important than family, friends, work, food, sex, anything. An addict may spend every waking hour trying to get or stay high. The disease can lie to him, making him forget the bad things that happen—the lows, the pain of withdrawal, the effects on his family. As one drug counselor put it, "If there are drugs behind you, your own son will run you over to get to them."[6] One social worker compared counseling an addict to "beating your head against a brick wall . . . because you are dealing with someone who has no control over her life. She's worried about her next hit."[7] Some young mothers have sold their baby's milk and diapers for drug money. Others sell their bodies, supporting their drug habit by becoming street prostitutes. As one former addict explained to a U.S. Senate committee, "Even though I wanted to quit, my need for the cocaine was greater than my maternal instinct."[8]

Addiction can also stunt a person's development. Pam Marshall sees it in her daughter. "It's frightening what it does to them," she says. "Once they start using the drug, they stop growing intellectually. Linda started using at 13, and her mind is still like a 13-year-old's. It's like she lost all the years in between." Another grandmother describes her adult son as "24 going on 14."

The behavior of an addict is controlled by drugs and alcohol. His behavior doesn't mean that your son doesn't love his children; her actions don't mean that your daughter is trying to hurt you. If your adult child doesn't seem at all like the child you raised, she probably isn't: drugs and alcohol have taken over her life.

■ WHAT YOU NEED TO KNOW

• *It's not your fault.* Pam Marshall remembers trying to explain her daughter's addiction to herself. "It was my fault," she says. "It was her father's fault. It was her peers' fault. You blame everyone and everything except the person herself. You look for excuses. You look back and try to figure out what happened, when it happened, how it happened . . . and you don't have any answers." There is no one answer for why a person drinks or takes drugs or why one person will become an addict and another one will not. But you are not to blame. You could raise four children and have only one of them turn to drugs. You could be an alcoholic yourself yet raise a family of staunch nondrinkers. Though you may never have touched a drop of wine, your child may be an alcoholic. We each make our own choices in life. Your children made theirs.

• *There is little you can do to help.* One of the most frustrating things for parents to accept is the fact that there is nothing they can do to *cure* their child of a drug or alcohol addiction. Remember, an addiction is a disease. You can't make it go away. Nor can you make your addicted child seek help. Certainly, you can drive your child to a treatment center or support group, but he is the one who must enter, stay, and participate. Too many parents pay for treatment after treatment when they are the ones who are motivated, not the addict.

If you want to facilitate treatment for your adult child, you can give her a list of programs in your area. You can watch her children while she is in rehabilitation. But if she is not ready to make her own appointment and show up for treatment, then it will only be an exercise in futility. The addict must be the one to recognize the problem and commit to seeking help.

All you can do is protect yourself and your grandchildren and try not to give in to your adult child's pleas and demands. An addict will use you, and you have to understand that. If you give an addicted child money, you finance his habit. You have to be strong enough both to love your child and to refuse him. It is the old rule of tough love (for more on tough love, see Chapter 5).

• *Recovery can be painfully slow.* Recovery from an alcohol or drug addiction is a long, complex process with no guaranteed results. Many people don't complete treatment programs, and the relapse rate is high. Even when addicts successfully complete a program, they are still at risk for returning to old habits. And they often can't tell you what happened or why. At one point, several grandparent families from GAP appeared on television.[9] Two of them were accompanied by their adult daughters, each of whom was in recovery and doing well. Unfortunately, a year later both daughters were back on the street. One was back in jail, where she gave birth to her fourth child. "The statistics for recovery are a lot like the statistics for weight loss programs," says one drug program coordinator. "How many people a year later have gained it back?"[10] Thus, getting into treatment is an important start, but there is still a long, frustrating fight ahead.

• *Seek emotional support.* If you have an adult child who is an addict, find a source of information and support. Al-Anon and Narc-Anon are 12-step groups for people who have relatives addicted to alcohol and drugs. Physicians, mental health professionals, and substance abuse counselors can help you understand what is happening to your child, and grandparent support groups can give you a forum where you can express feelings and frustrations and receive reassurance that your feelings and concerns are normal. Don't try to weather your child's addiction alone; find a source of emotional support and use it often.

• *Release hope . . .* It sounds strange to say, but sometimes the kindest thing you can do for yourself is to release your grip on hope. Hope keeps you paying for treatment after treatment, looking for the magic one. Hope keeps you and your grandchildren waiting at the door imagining that this time Mom or Dad will be sober and committed to abstinence. The truth is that your son or daughter may—or may not—recover. But the battle is not yours. You cannot make your child better; it is not in your control. "You never really *give up* hope," says one grandmother. "You don't give up on your kids. But you do decide to give up the chaos, to be strong enough not to allow them to come into your home, your life, your grandchild's life and cause drama. We have enough battles; we don't have to fight them, too."

- ... *but expect anything.* Despite all the doom and gloom predictions, some people do recover. Something in them is resilient enough to fight back and win. Sometimes the most unlikely candidate for success will surprise you. Take the story of Dorsey Nunn, a prisoners' rights advocate in San Francisco. A recovered addict himself, he took in his nephews when his mother died. "I'm sure Mom didn't recognize when I was serving a life sentence that I'd be the one raising the family," says Nunn. "You can look for hope in the most unlikely circumstances. Besides, if no one advocates for recovery, grandparents will be raising grandchildren for a long time to come."[11]

YOUR DRUG-EXPOSED GRANDCHILDREN

Katherine Connor hardly slept at all the first five months after her third granddaughter arrived. Because the drug-exposed baby had a tendency to stop breathing at night, Katherine slept at the foot of her own bed, propped high on pillows so she could look down into the crib. Her clothes laid out nearby, Grandma was ready to run to the hospital if she had to. As Becky got older, Katherine finally got to sleep for intervals of three to four hours.

Baby Jay was also born with drugs in his system. He could barely breathe, his body was unusually rigid, and the doctors thought he might never walk. When she first saw him, says his grandmother, "He was frantic. His little eyes darted from side to side. His tongue came out like a serpent's tongue. You knew he had problems." When he first came home from the hospital, Jay went through four months of "withdrawal," shaking and crying uncontrollably. One weekend he screamed for 52 hours straight. Sometimes his grandparents would float him in warm water to calm him down; then they would swaddle him tight in a blanket and rock him through it.

Sue Campbell feels lucky. Although her daughter Rachel was a 20-year addict, her granddaughter Mandi was born free of drugs in her system. "My miracle baby," Sue calls her. Still, she doesn't know what could happen 10 years down the line. There is too little information about the long-term effects of prenatal drug exposure for Sue to feel completely safe that Mandi is in the clear, and she continues to watch her granddaughter closely.

It's hard to know exactly how many newborns are exposed to drugs and alcohol in the womb. Some studies estimate that 1 in every 10 newborns is exposed in the womb to one or more illicit drugs.[12] However, not all states require health care professionals to test for prenatal drug exposure,[13] and some toxicology screens can only identify drug use within the previous 24 to 72 hours, depending on the drug.[14]

Whatever the statistics, the result of a pregnant woman's addiction can be heartrending: an underweight infant, shaking and crying; an underdeveloped toddler; an older child who shows a range of difficulties from learning disabilities to emotional and behavioral problems. For grandparents, unprepared to raise a second family, drug-exposed children are an exhausting challenge.

The following paragraphs discuss what you need to know about drug-exposed children: the symptoms and risks of prenatal drug exposure for children; the special demands on you as caregivers (for example, the late-night vigils ahead of you); and recommendations from experts and other grandparents on how to handle common issues like tremors and uncontrollable crying. Understand, however, that no one can present an exact picture of how a drug-exposed child will look or act. There is no formula, no equation, to guide you. Much depends on what substances the mother took, how much of them she took, and at what point in the pregnancy she took them.

Nor does every child react to drug exposure equally. Some children may exhibit many symptoms whereas others may not experience any. Some children may have difficulties that only appear as they get older. Although the outcome of prenatal drug exposure can vary from one infant to another, all babies born to substance-abusing mothers are at risk for developmental, learning, and behavioral problems, as well as for fragile physical health.

The symptoms and risks discussed in this chapter are only generalizations. They are not included to scare you but to keep you aware of the possibilities. Try not to look for trouble, but, at the same time, keep your eyes open for the small signs that suggest that your grandchild might require extra help. The earlier you catch problems, the sooner you can address them.

Drug-Exposed Infants

The first few days after delivery can be quite an ordeal for infants born with drugs present in their systems and for the people who care for them. The babies go through a process similar to chemical withdrawal, which can include tremors, seizures, and uncontrollable crying. They can be frustrating to care for, since they do not respond to many of the cues normal infants respond to, like bouncing and cooing (in fact, some will even arch their backs to get away). The stress of this period means that a drug-exposed infant can miss out on some of the early weeks of learning and bonding, which are so important to a child's emotional development. Once any actual drugs are gone from the baby's system, there can still be physical and psychological ramifications from the prenatal drug exposure, as well as possible medical risks.

Drug-Exposed Toddlers and Children

Children of substance-abusing mothers are at risk for a number of challenges as they grow up. Respiratory and neurological problems, visual and hearing deficits, birth defects, cerebral palsy, and mental retardation are not uncommon in drug-exposed children, although not every such child will have medical complications. Some of these children may have difficulty with motor development; their hands may shake when they reach for objects, and they could have trouble learning to walk. Some may be slow in learning to talk or in completing toilet training. They may be easily stimulated and may show an inclination toward hyperactive and impulsive behavior. They may have difficulty paying attention, which can cause problems when they start school. In fact, many drug-exposed children

Is Your Grandbaby Drug Exposed?

It is easy to tell if your grandchild was exposed to drugs in the womb if the infant tests positive for unprescribed medication or drugs in his or her system at birth. Unfortunately, some toxicology screens only show drug use within the previous 24- to 72-hour period. This means that a fetus can be exposed to drugs and alcohol for months before delivery and these substances may not show up in his or her system if the mother abstained from chemical abuse during the week before delivery. If that was the case with your grandchild, prenatal drug exposure is a puzzle you and your doctor must piece together from a variety of clues.

The following signs may indicate prenatal drug exposure in an infant if several are present and not due to some other medical condition. If you suspect your grandchild was exposed to drugs in the womb, contact a physician.

- Premature birth
- Low birth weight
- Small head
- Seemingly constant shaking or trembling
- Difficulty feeding
- High-pitched, inconsolable cry
- Difficult to comfort
- Seizures
- Is unresponsive and lethargic
- Diarrhea
- Vomiting
- Frantic sucking
- Stiff, rigid body
- Staring or unusual eye movements
- Irregular breathing pattern
- Startle response to the least sound or touch
- Easily overstimulated
- Sleeps too much
- Doesn't sleep at all
- Physical signs of fetal alcohol syndrome (FAS), such as small, widely spaced eyes, small, flat cheeks, and a short, upturned nose

exhibit symptoms of attention-deficit/hyperactivity disorder (ADHD) and various learning disabilities. However, each of these conditions has been associated with many different outcomes. Whether a condition becomes a handicap or a challenge has a lot to do with how a child is helped and how his or her needs are met.

It is important to understand that the effect of drug exposure is unpredictable. There is no typical drug-exposed infant or child. Not all babies exposed to drugs and alcohol suffer equally. Some children may be obviously affected by their mother's addiction: Like Becky, they may be premature and medically fragile. Like Jay, they may suffer through symptoms of withdrawal. They may have the facial characteristics often associated with fetal alcohol syndrome (FAS). Some children may not seem to be affected at all; they may look and act just like other children, but learning and/or behavioral problems may show up in preschool, kindergarten, or even later. Others, surprisingly, may completely escape harm.

How an individual child is affected can depend on what the mother used and when in the pregnancy she used it. It can depend on her health and nutrition and on whether or not she received prenatal care. It can depend on the temperament of the individual child. It might also be a question of luck. We just don't know enough yet to predict.

But while substance abuse by the mother doesn't guarantee damage to the infant, all children born to substance-abusing mothers are *at risk* for problems as they grow up.

▦ HOW TO COPE

• *Reduce stimulation.* Many drug-exposed infants are easily stimulated and difficult to calm. This can be particularly troublesome when you're trying to get the child to sleep. If your grandchild is an overly excitable baby, consider reducing the outside stimulation in the environment. Try to eliminate loud noises, bright lights, sudden movements. This is hard to do with other children in the house, but do as much as you can. Consider what you have on the walls and in the crib. Is it bright and distracting? Can you keep lights low? Can you turn off the television? Speak to the baby in a soft voice, or hum and rock to soothe him. Don't handle or jiggle the baby too much, and try not to do too many things at once, even soothing things. It will just rev him up all over again.

• *Try swaddling.* Two of the symptoms of a drug-exposed infant are a prolonged, piercing cry and uncontrollable shaking. Unlike normal babies, who cry but eventually fall asleep, drug-exposed infants are unable to calm themselves and will continue to cry and shake and flail their arms and legs. Your first instinct might be to rock the baby or to pace with or bounce her up and down as you whisper soothing sounds. Unfortunately, these things only add to the stimulation. Try swaddling instead. Wrap her snugly in a blanket and hold her close to your body. Soothing the baby in this way cuts down on her own activity and reduces the stimulation. "You wrap them close to you and let them feel your heart," says Katherine Connor. "It's like kittens with a clock."

Never swaddle a baby who has a fever or trouble breathing.

• *Be vigilant.* Raising any child requires you to be constantly alert to signs of illness or sounds of trouble. Drug-exposed children demand twice as much vigilance, since they may be medically fragile as infants and hyperactive as toddlers. "You need to watch these babies during the night," says Alice Sutherland, a former pediatric nurse who is raising two drug-exposed grandchildren. "They have a lot of problems in the first years. You have to stay alert. You don't sleep soundly, or you're going to lose them. You need to monitor them and go into that room and actually feel them."

Once drug-exposed children start walking, the issues change. You can't assume that the child is still in bed or that the child gate is still keeping her out of danger. The question is not "How is the child?" but "Where is the child?" "These are not dumb children," says Alice. "You have to outthink them. When it's quiet, think, 'Why is it quiet?' And find them quickly."

• *Learn about these children.* If you know or suspect that your grandchild is drug-exposed, educate yourself. Talk to doctors, experts, and grandparents who have been where you are now. The more you know about the effects of drug exposure, the earlier you can address any difficulties your grandchild may have, whether they involve a hearing deficit, a language delay, or poor motor control. If you suspect any kind of problem, take preventive measures. Get your grandchild a thorough physical.

• *Look into early intervention.* Every state offers early intervention programs to address developmental and learning disabilities before children enter the school system. Some states even provide services to infants and toddlers. If you think your grandchild could benefit from early intervention, contact your state board of education and ask which department handles such programs. (For more on early intervention, see Chapter 13.)

• *Find outside support.* A drug-exposed infant can make you feel like a failure. Many of the things you did to soothe and care for your own babies may not work with this one, and you may not know why. Still, many grandparents are reluctant to admit they don't know what they're doing and are shy about asking for help. Don't suffer in silence; look for support. There are many local and national organizations that can provide free information on caring for drug-exposed children. Grandparent support groups are also a wonderful source of advice and support. Not only do they offer you a forum to express your frustration, but they are a place to hear other grandparents' experiences and the solutions they found.

• *Avoid the dangers of labels.* Just because a child was exposed to drugs does not mean that he is doomed by them. Remember, the effects of drug exposure are unpredictable. Moreover, many of the symptoms that drug-exposed infants experience are similar to those of premature infants who were not exposed to drugs or alcohol in the womb.

The trouble with labels is that they can limit our understanding of an individual child. If relatives, teachers, or physicians focus too closely on the fact that a child's mother was an addict, they run the danger of assuming that all the child's problems are caused by prenatal drugs and may not consider other possibilities, such as heredity, disease, or emotional distress. One baby kept returning to the hospital with what everyone thought were seizures; now the doctors believe he was suffering from frequent ear infections. Labels can also create self-fulfilling prophecies. If you expect a child to fail, he probably will.

If your grandchild was exposed to drugs in the womb, definitely watch for related symptoms. But watch for all kinds of symptoms—just as you would with any child. Don't let anyone dismiss your grandchild as a "drug child" without asking deeper questions.

• *Know your grandchild's family medical history.* As more and more medical conditions are proving to be hereditary, it is difficult to overemphasize the importance of a family medical history. Respiratory problems can certainly be related to drug exposure, but they can also be inherited. Hyperactivity is also believed to be a genetic condition. Poor feeding can be signs of an allergy to milk. The more you can find out about your grandchild's family background, the better you can help your pediatrician attend to the child's needs. Even if the child is placed with you from a foster home, ask for all available medical records or medical history.

• *Don't lose hope.* Prenatal drug exposure can be a serious medical and developmental challenge for a child, but it doesn't have to be a sentence to failure. The jury is still out on the long-term physical and psychological effects, and some early studies indicate that with proper intervention there is reason to hope for a good outcome in many cases. In fact, some experts predict that many children prenatally exposed to drugs and alcohol can develop into healthy children and responsible members of the community. "This is not a lost generation," says one inner-city pediatrician. "These children are not monsters. They are salvageable, capable of loving, of making good attachments. Yes, they present problems that we have not dealt with before, but they can be taught."[15]

Alice Sutherland knows the truth of that statement. All three of her grandchildren were born drug exposed, and she has seen them make great strides in their development. When the oldest was struggling in public school, Alice put her in a magnet school for the performing arts, hoping the child's love of music would give her motivation. Sarah is still only an average student, but at age 13, she has already appeared in a television commercial and hopes to be an actress someday. "Success," says Alice, "all depends on the person raising the child. The drug is just a medical problem the first five or so years. Intellectually, these children are very intelligent. You watch; you'll see all individual people."

• *Love, love, love them.* Children learn to trust the world when they have consistent and responsive caregivers who accept them as they are and who provide them with a safe environment in which to strive. The more they trust their immediate world, the more they trust themselves to try new things. If there is any medicine that is guaranteed to work wonders on your grandchild, it is your love. It's the secret ingredient every grandmother knows:

> "You're going to have to know that your life stops on a dime," says Fay Strassburger. "The only thing that exists at that time is that baby, because that baby needs all the attention, all the love and all the caring you can possibly give him."[16]

"They thrive on that," says Alice Sutherland. "That's what gets them through—knowing they are secure and that there's a lot of love."

"This is love," says Katherine Connor. "That's the key to why my babies are all surviving; they know they have a grandma who loves them."

STOPPING THE CYCLE: RAISING THE NEXT GENERATION

At 15, Jessica Hulsey was already a crusader against drugs. The daughter of addicted parents, the California teenager knew firsthand what drugs did to a family and to a child, and had spoken out against them in compositions, school assemblies, and newspaper articles. "I missed a lot," she told the *Orange County Register.* "I grew up so fast, and I had to worry about my sister and family. I will never forgive drugs for taking [normal life] away from me."[17] By the time she turned 21, Jessica was a nationally recognized advocate for drug prevention and a member of the President's Commission on Drug-Free Communities.[18]

While they may not all be as vocal as Jessica, many children of addicted parents harbor intense negative feelings about drugs and alcohol. They have seen what it does, and they swear they want no part of it. It's the kind of statement that fills a grandparent's heart with relief.

Unfortunately, however sweet they are, declarations and promises are not guarantees. Don't let them lull you into looking the other way. The sad fact is that children of alcohol and drug abusers run a high risk of using drugs and alcohol themselves. The combination of peer pressure and curiosity about drugs and alcohol can be overwhelming to teenagers and children. It is estimated that 75 percent of all high school students have tried alcohol, tobacco, or some kind of legal or illicit drugs, and 20 percent of those teens are addicted.[19] Your challenge, then, becomes how to prevent an at-risk grandchild from becoming an at-risk teenager. While there is no foolproof way to keep a child off drugs, there are some precautions you can take:

• *Accept the possibility.* "Not my child." Those are the three words that get a parent, or grandparent, into the most trouble when it comes to drugs and alcohol. They keep you from watching for changed or strange behavior, they keep you from asking questions and finding help, and they offer you false hope. The truth is that any child may bend to peer pressure and curiosity. The only way to stop the cycle of drug and alcohol abuse is to understand that it is a cycle and that your grandchild may be at risk for addictive behavior. Don't bury your head in the sand. If a grandchild's behavior seems suspicious, ask questions.

• *Teach your grandchildren to say no to drugs.* If your grandchildren are old enough to understand, talk to them about drugs. If you have already discussed the subject in talking about their parents, continue the conversation. It is not enough to teach them to refuse drugs; they have to know why, and your best examples may be close to home. Provide them with clear, factual information about all mind-altering substances. Remember that street drugs are not the only danger. Over 2,000 teenagers a day experiment with pain relievers for the first time.[20] Prescription drugs and OTC medications like cough and cold remedies can be just as dangerous as illegal drugs when misused. Nurture your grandchildren's self-esteem and discuss different ways of handling peer pressure. A child who is prepared to say no may have an easier time actually saying it.

• *Be a good role model.* Set clear rules about drugs and medications. Teach your grandchildren never to share prescriptions and to follow proper dosages. Make sure you follow the same rules yourself. And look at your own use of alcohol and tobacco: what messages are you sending?

• *Monitor the medicine cabinet.* Keep prescription and OTC medications in a secure place and control access to it. Keep track of quantities, and make sure to properly dispose of expired or unused medication. Again, educate your grandkids about the dangers of these drugs, just as you would the dangers of household poisons. And ask family and friends to safeguard their medicine cabinets as well.

• *Supervise your grandchildren.* The best way to know what is happening in your grandchildren's lives is to be actively involved in them. Know their friends and their interests. Be aware of where they go and whom they're with. Don't allow your involvement in their lives to deteriorate into an inquisition but maintain it as a normal part of your relationship. Not only will you be aware of changes in their lives, but you may build a closer, more trusting relationship with them.

• *Learn to recognize drug use.* Unlike childhood diseases like mumps and measles, drug abuse does not always have overt physical symptoms. However, there are warning signs a grandparent can watch for, if you know enough to look. They are the same signs many grandparents innocently tossed off as "growing pains," "teenage changes," and "the flu" when they were raising their own children: changes in eating and sleeping patterns, restlessness, sudden sulking or excessive energy. The accompanying box lists some of the symptoms of teen drug use. Familiarize yourself with them and stay active in your grandchild's life; if the changes are there, you will then be in the best position to spot them.

Don't be paranoid, however. It can be difficult to know the difference between erratic but normal behavior in kids and behavior caused by drugs. Every change is not an alarm. The changes to be concerned about are those that seem severe or that last more than a few days. Even if they are not linked to drug use, changes could signal medical problems, depression, or trouble at home or at school. If you do suspect anything, seek professional help.

• *Seek outside help.* Drug information alone may not be enough to keep a child off drugs. Self-esteem, positive role models, and peer support are also important. Schools and youth groups often sponsor antidrug programs. There are also many national and local organizations that offer resources to help you help your grandchild stay drug free. Search under "drug-free kids" for groups in your area.

Could Your Grandchild Be Using Drugs or Alcohol?

The Warning Signs

Although experimenting with drugs and alcohol has almost become a rite of passage with teenagers, many children don't limit themselves to curious experiments. Instead, they slip down the steep path to habit and addiction.

Has your grandchild:

- Become hostile or uncooperative?
- Become withdrawn and depressed?

(cont.)

Could Your Grandchild Be Using Drugs or Alcohol? (*cont.*)

- Suddenly dropped old friends?
- Become careless about his or her appearance?
- Lost interest in favorite hobbies or sports?

Is your grandchild:

- Suddenly doing poorly in school?
- Skipping classes?
- Borrowing money without a clear explanation?
- Experiencing unexplained bursts of energy?
- Experiencing a severe weight loss?
- Experiencing a change in eating or sleeping patterns?
- Unresponsive or aggressive with family members?

Does your grandchild seem:

- Constantly tired?
- Forgetful?
- Restless?
- Excessively talkative?
- Irrational?
- Clumsy?
- Drunk or spacey?

Many of these symptoms could be warning signs of excessive use of drugs or alcohol, as are dilated or pinpoint pupils, flushed skin, needle marks, and the presence of drug paraphernalia like needles, water pipes, pills, and roach clips.

Many of these symptoms are not limited to drug use; they can also indicate depression, an eating disorder, or some other psychological or medical problem. Whatever their cause, they warrant investigation.

A FINAL WORD

The information in this chapter has presented only some of the possible outcomes for drug-exposed children. Many of these outcomes can be frightening to consider, but they are only generalizations. They are described here to help you keep your eyes open, not to cause despair. Your grandchildren's lives are still being written. If anything will give them the chance to succeed, it is your love and patience in raising them.

9

When Parents Get Their Children Back

What makes me scared is that my mom could take me anytime she wants. I always told myself if she does come and try to get me, I plan to run away. I'm not going to lead that hellish life.

—Cameron, age 15

Grandma's house was a safe house for Marjorie Brown's two grandchildren. Jessica, age three, arrived at the age of six months with fingernail marks up and down her back and a huge bruise on one leg. Her mother, Valerie, told Marjorie to take Jessica before she hurt her even more. Billy came almost a year later, when child protective services removed him from his mother because of neglect. Valerie, a drug addict who had been involved with gangs since she was 14, had been in and out of jail on several counts and had only seen Billy four times in eight months. She had not complied with court-ordered counseling or drug programs and was not allowed to see her children without another adult present. Even Valerie's parole officer described her as a "walking time bomb." When the unthinkable happened and a juvenile court judge decided Valerie was ready to parent and ordered Billy back to his mother, Marjorie was floored. In her wildest imaginings, she hadn't expected this. She knew Valerie couldn't handle the baby. The social worker knew it. Even Valerie knew she wasn't ready for full-time motherhood—and said so. However, the judge, noting that Valerie had had several clean drug tests and that she wanted unmonitored visits, decided she was ready.

Today, Marjorie and Valerie have a voluntary arrangement. Billy lives with Marjorie, but Valerie can take him whenever and wherever she likes. Marjorie is scared to death. She sees Valerie driving around with gang members and dressing like one; she worries that her daughter is using drugs again. She is afraid of drive-by shootings with the baby in the car. Mostly, she is afraid of her daughter's temper. "Billy's at the point where he's walking and getting into things," she says. "Valerie has already expressed that she couldn't handle him, and she'd only had him twenty-four hours. She couldn't take the stress of his screaming. I'm afraid she's going to hurt him. If she could hurt Jessica at six months, what could she do to Billy?"

In addition to her own fears, Marjorie is having problems with Jessica. Jessica's court case is separate from her brother's, and she is not legally affected by the judge's decision. Nevertheless, the emotional toll on the little girl has been heavy. She had begun to open up and play with other children; now she is withdrawn and is having nightmares. She sees her mother taking Billy, and she is terrified that she will have to go with her, too. "She wakes up in the night screaming, 'I don't want to go with Valerie!'" says Marjorie. "I hold her and tell her she is not going, but she sees Billy come and go, and she doesn't know what to make of it. She used to love to go to McDonald's. That's our meeting place now. She won't eat at McDonald's anymore. That's pretty bad, when a child doesn't want to eat at McDonald's."

Sending children back to their parents can be a grandparent's fondest dream—and worst nightmare. The dream is that the adult children will shape up and become active, responsible parents, that the grandchildren will be safe, and that you can resume your role of occasional babysitter and doting grandparent. The nightmare is that the children will go back before the parents have their lives in order, before it is truly safe.

For some grandparents, dreams do come true. There are parents who hit a bad patch in their lives and come out of it. There are addicts and alcoholics who recover and resume normal lives. Unfortunately, there are also many grandparents who wake up to discover the nightmares are real: A mother who hasn't seen a child in three years shows up and wants him back; an absent father remarries and suddenly wants his children; and the court decides that the parents are ready to take their children again, although, as far as the grandparents know, they are still using drugs. Nothing can prevent the shock and heartache of sending a child back to potentially unfit parents. Even when you know it can happen, you don't want to believe that it will. But when you don't see it coming, the pain is that much deeper.

FOREWARNED AND FOREARMED

The truth is that unless you have adopted your grandchildren or the parents are dead, you are at risk of losing them. If you have the children on an informal basis, the parents have every right to take them, even after several years. If they have been placed with you through the dependency system, you should be aware that the court's goal is to reunify children with their parents and that everything will be done to accomplish that. Even if you have private legal guardianship, it can be overturned if the parents prove themselves fit (although this puts the burden on the parent and is less likely). Neither you nor your grandchild is protected from the parent's ultimate right to parent, and you need to be prepared for anything, particularly when you deal with the juvenile court. Knowing these facts won't lessen the pain if you lose your grandchildren, but it can help you prepare for the worst.

Remember, you may have little control over what happens to your grandchildren tomorrow, but you have a lot of control over what happens today. You can give your grandchildren the best care you can while you have them. You can give them a foundation of love and self-esteem. If they are old enough, you can teach them the skills they need to take care of themselves—simple things like how to call 911, how to make a peanut butter sandwich, how to call you collect. One grandmother taught her twins her phone number by inventing a song. You can also make sure they know that certain kinds of spanking and touching are not okay and that they should talk to a trusted adult if anything like that ever happens, even while they are living with you.

IF THE UNIMAGINABLE HAPPENS

If you do have to give up your grandchildren, you will feel like your heart has been torn out. Your life will be turned upside down yet again. You will have traveled the road from grandparent to parent; reorganized your life around these children; and loved and nurtured them for months, if not years, and now you will be expected to give them back like any part-time baby-sitter. It's hard, and it's painful. All the complex feelings you went through when your grandchildren first arrived may double back on you with a vengeance. But now there may be new layers: guilty thoughts that if you had handled something differently, they might still be with you; false hopes that maybe your adult child really can get it together this time; renewed rage at the system and the parents; uncertainty over if and when you will see your grandchildren again; fear for their safety; and a feeling of deep helplessness over your inability to protect them. It can feel like there is a huge void where your heart should be. You might find yourself distancing from them, if only to protect yourself.

Your grandchildren will have their own mixed reactions to going back to their parents. They may repeat behaviors that you thought were long behind them: bed-wetting, explosions of anger, school problems. Children who don't want to leave you may feel like you're sending them away; they may regress or push you away, or they may misbehave, hoping that if they're bad enough, their parents won't want them. Children who want to be with Mom or Dad may stop listening to you once they know they're going home. They, too, might misbehave, thinking that if you've had enough, you'll send them sooner. They may be caught between conflicting feelings and may express them in angry outbursts.

Either way, your grandchildren will be uprooted again and will need help with the transition. If you are lucky, you will have time to prepare them. You can reassure them that you are not sending them away and that you'll try to keep in contact. Although you can't speak for what Mom or Dad will allow—parents may lie to their children about allowing them to see you—you can promise your grandchildren that if you can't see them, you will think about them and continue to love them. Children who start acting out behaviorally will need help putting their feelings into words. If they are in counseling, they need to focus on this change. Also, let teachers know what is happening so that they can help, too.

Sometimes, however, you won't have the luxury of transition time. The judge in Marjorie's case would have let Mom take the baby directly from the courtroom, with no transition at all, except that Valerie herself objected. If this happens, all you can do is give yourself room to grieve.

If, like Marjorie, you have other grandchildren at home, you will also have to deal with their reactions: fear that they, too, might have to leave; anger at being left behind; sorrow at being separated from their siblings; or fear for their siblings and concern that they may never see them again. All you can do is reassure them that you love them, that you understand their feelings, and that for now they are safe with you. Unfortunately, it is the man in the robe who is making the decisions.

Then there are the practical issues. What do you send with the children? Do you give Mom all the baby's things? Certainly, you want the child to have them, but will that be the case? Or will Mom sell the high chair for drug money? And what if Mom can't parent two months from now, and the kids come back to you? Won't you need a high chair and car seat? My recommendation is to play it by ear. Everything depends on your individual history with the parent. Do whatever you are comfortable doing. Perhaps you can give a few things at a time and see what happens. Look at the whole picture before you decide what, and how much, to give away.

OUT OF SIGHT, OUT OF REACH

Perhaps the hardest thing for a grandparent to face in this situation is the wrath of the parent who believes you "stole" the children (even if it was child protective services that removed them in the first place). Parent–grandparent relationships will be strained at best and can escalate to outright hostility. In the worst cases, parents deny grandparents all access to the grandchildren.

A Wisconsin grandmother had to spend close to $30,000 in attorney fees just to get one monthly visit and one weekly phone call with a granddaughter she had raised for nine years. A Minnesota grandfather used to go to his grandsons' school to watch them play ball, but Mom got a restraining order so that he can't even do that anymore. These grandparents send cards and gifts without knowing if they are received. Some are returned. They have lost grandchildren not only from their homes but also from their lives.

■ HOW TO COPE

When your grandchildren go back, it can feel like the world has ended and the nightmare has begun. Nothing will take the pain away, but there are some things you can do to help yourself adjust.

• *Give yourself time to grieve.* Your sadness, your anger, and the huge sense of emptiness are normal. You have suffered an enormous loss, and you need to process your feelings in a safe, comfortable way. This is a time to seek out support. If friends and family are too overwhelmed, consider counseling. And definitely seek out support groups. Just because you no longer have your grandchildren doesn't mean you are barred from grandparent groups. If anything, this is a time when you most need to be with people who understand the depth of your loss.

• *Try to move on.* It sounds cold, but there's not much you can do once a judge has decided that a parent is rehabilitated. Whatever is going to happen will happen. Perhaps the parent *has* pulled herself together. If not, maybe the child will end up back in the system, and they'll call you. But you can't put your life on hold until then, and it won't help your grandchild if you do.

• *Get busy.* Spend time with your other grandchildren; they also need you in their lives. Volunteer. Some grandparents have found it helpful to volunteer in a hospital or a school when they miss being around kids. Get involved with all the hobbies you put on hold. Spend more time with people you care about—your spouse, family, and friends.

• *Get politically involved.* Many grandparents at the forefront of the grandparents' movement have channeled their grief and anger into activism. They may not be able to help their own grandchildren, they reason, but they can fight to prevent other grandchildren and grandparents from suffering similar traumas. One of the hardest things to accept as a grandparent is how helpless you are in the system; political action offers you a chance to affect the system and empower yourself in the process.

THE NEVER-ENDING CYCLE

Two of Sandra Cobb's seven grandchildren were returned to a mother who swore she was off drugs. She tested clean, met regularly with her probation officer, had a steady job, and appeared to be ready to care for two babies. It didn't last. Several months later, Mom resumed her drug use, lost her job, and started prostituting herself again. When she left the boys alone in her apartment, a neighbor called the police. The children were taken into protective custody and given back to Grandma.

When you are returning your grandchildren to their parents, it is cold comfort to think that they might soon be back. It means that they will have been mistreated again and that they will return to you with emotional wounds reopened. It is rare that children go home to Mom and Dad and actually stay with them. Another truth about these adult children is that they rarely pull it together for long. They go into rehab. They get jobs. They even stay clean for one or two years—long enough to impress a judge and raise your hopes. But they walk a thin line between good intentions and immediate gratification, and they are prone to misstep.

After years of self-protection, Pam and Robert Marshall finally allowed themselves some hope. Linda had been clean nearly two years. She had a job and an apartment. She started to show more than a passing interest in her daughter, calling and visiting more often, and she started talking about a future for herself. Then something snapped. She started using drugs again. She got pregnant and hooked up with an abusive ex-boyfriend whom she tracked down in jail. Now she's back in rehab, and her parents are devastated.

Even as you grieve the new loss of your grandchildren, brace yourself for anything. This, too, could be temporary. If you are allowed to see the children, keep a close eye on them. Try to stay on the parent's good side, even if it means walking on eggshells to do it. Offer to baby-sit. Above all, continue to document. Even if you are barred from seeing your grandchildren, keep a log. Whenever you make a call or send a card, even if the parent interferes with your attempt, write it down. If you can, find some way of knowing where your grandchildren are and how they are. If they are removed again—and they very well may be—you need to know about it.

AGAINST ALL ODDS

Melanie Waters moved from Chicago to Michigan to raise her three grandsons. Her daughter was on every drug she could get her hands on, and Melanie obtained legal guardianship in order to keep the boys out of crack houses. After a painful cycle of rehab and relapse, Grace disappeared completely. "I knew, as a mother, that she was gone," says Melanie. "I knew nothing I was going to do would change her destiny."

Marcia and Peter Weiss had two-year-old Max and his mom living with them when Heidi decided she couldn't take it anymore. She hooked up with a drug addict and skinhead, fully tattooed with swastikas, which was particularly hard on her Jewish parents. Heidi wasn't on drugs herself, but Marcia almost wishes she had been. "It would have justified her abandoning Max," she explains.

Rita Ward already had guardianship of one granddaughter when the call came from the hospital. Her drug-addict daughter had just lost custody of the toddler and the newborn. Would she take them?

These sound like three more horror stories from the kinship files—three more grandmothers who had to give up hope to protect their grandchildren. Except that something here was different, something that no one could ever predict or plan for: hope came and found them. It didn't happen at once, and it didn't happen easily, but against all odds, their adult children got their lives together. In each case, it felt like a miracle:

Grace had been missing for three years when Melanie took a business trip to Chicago. She was looking for a parking space and wondering, still, if she would ever see her daughter again, when there, walking across the street, was Grace. Like something out of a movie, they fell crying into each other's arms. Grace had been living on the streets, stoned and turning tricks, with no perception of time passing until an abscess put her in the hospital and she nearly died. The day she was released, a street minister asked if he could pray for her. "I want to find my mom and my kids," she told him. The next day, she walked in front of Melanie's car. She began a rigorous process of healing and rehab in Chicago, stabilized, and finally moved to Michigan to be with Melanie and the boys. It wasn't an easy transition. The kids were used to Grandma's rules, and there were resentments to work through. "You're going to have to find your relationships yourself," Melanie told her. And slowly, they have. Today Melanie and Grace are still living together and learning to co-parent. "There is hope," says Melanie. "You never know when angels are going to show up."

The worst thing Marcia and Peter could have imagined was their daughter's skinhead boyfriend as a son-in-law, and they were relieved that Heidi never brought him when she visited Max. But Craig surprised them by getting sober and by having his tattoos removed. When Max was six, Heidi married Craig, with both of her parents in attendance. Getting physical custody of Max was a slower process. Marcia and Peter never relinquished their guardianship status, but they drew up a legal agreement specifying how reunification might happen. Little by little, they gave the younger couple more childrearing privileges, and by the time Max was eight, Heidi and Craig had full parenting responsibilities. Craig has turned out to be a great stepdad, and Marcia and Peter are thrilled to be Grandma and Grandpa again. "Heidi was always nurturing," says Marcia. "So to see her abandon her baby was a shock. Now the relationship is what it might have been if that hadn't happened."

Rita had continued to have a good rapport with Kate, despite her addiction. Then one day, Kate vanished from rehab and hit the streets again. She had been living in a family rental property outside Pittsburgh, and Rita didn't think she'd come back, so she rented out the apartment. When Kate resurfaced, she was angry and resentful. She blamed Rita for kicking her out. But it turned out to be the best thing that could have happened. By the time the youngest was two, Kate was clean and sober. She regained custody of the younger girls and slowly began to repair her relationship with the oldest, who remained with Rita. Sixteen years later, Kate is still clean. "My daughter has turned out to be a fabulous mother," says Rita with pride. "And the baby I got out of the hospital just turned 18."

By this point, you are probably reading these stories like tea leaves, looking for clues that will turn a hopeless story into one of hope. I hate to say it, but it can't be done. Or rather, *you* can't do it. Just as no one knows what turns one person into an addict or an abusive parent, no one knows why one person recovers and another doesn't. Each adult child takes a unique path into chaos, and each must find an individual path out. You have to be realists, I often tell grandparents. But as David Ben-Gurion once said, "In order to be a realist, you must believe in miracles." These families shared their stories to remind you that miracles do happen. That sometimes the light at the end of the tunnel is not a rushing train, but a new tomorrow. That some families do heal.

SECTION II

Through the Red Tape

10
Grandparenting and the Law

Never to such an extent in U.S. history has care of children by relatives been so interwoven with government.
—*Newsletter of the National Association of Court-Appointed Special Advocates for Children*[1]

I f you are a grandparent raising a grandchild, the odds are good that at some point you will end up in a courtroom. The process could be as simple as filing for guardianship with the parent's consent, or it could be as heartrending as a fight to keep your grandchild from being returned to an abusive home. Either way, many strangers—judges, social workers, and attorneys—will have a say in determining what happens to your family. Even if you are not actually raising your grandchildren, you could find yourself rubbing shoulders with the law. The divorce rate is approximately one out of every two marriages, and sometimes grandparents have to petition the courts to be able to see their grandchildren.

Many grandparents have gone their entire lives without entering a court of law. They may think that litigation, like violence, is something that happens to other people—those in the newspapers or on television. But they do believe in justice, and they expect it to be there when they need it. Then they enter the legal system and discover that judicial proceedings can be confusing, impersonal, and often expensive, both financially and emotionally. The cost can affect your bank account and your spirit. The process is painfully slow. And the underlying principles don't always feel friendly to grandparents, even though a number of federal and state laws have formally acknowledged the importance of extended family in the lives of children.

This book cannot change the realities of the legal system, but it can attempt to clear up some of the confusion. This chapter and the next are designed as road maps of the key legal issues you may encounter with your grandchildren, namely, your rights as a grandparent, possible custody arrangements, and the landmarks of the juvenile dependency system. They are designed to give you enough information to ask informed questions. Knowledge is power, and the best protection you have is an understanding of the terrain. First, however, a few warnings:

• *The legal system is complex and changeable.* While laws are spelled out, interpretations are not. Everything in court depends on the facts of the individual case and the interpretation of the individual judge. To quote one family court judge, "I can't say, 'This is the law, and if you connect the five following dots, you win.'" Law is never that simple, and legislation may change over time.

• *Family and children's issues are handled in a variety of different courts.* There is no one-stop shop when families interact with the law. Instead, there is a roster of individual courts—family, probate, adoptions, and juvenile—that interpret the law in regard to a range of issues, from divorce, child custody, visitation, guardianship, and adoption to juvenile delinquency, juvenile dependency, and foster care.

• *A courtroom has a unique culture.* Attorneys and courts use legal terms, shorthand, jargon, and abbreviations. They speak a different language, and they're talking about things that have far-reaching consequences for your grandchild and your family.

• *Most family issues are governed by state, not federal, legislation.* This means that laws and regulations about marriage, divorce, paternity, visitation, guardianship, and adoption can vary from state to state, as can legal definitions and standards of proof. And while dependency proceedings are guided by federal legislation, certain timelines and regulations may vary by state. Even basic terminology is location-driven. What is called probate court in California is surrogate's court in New York. "Visitation" in one state may be "access" or "parental contact" somewhere else. "Guardianship" may be "managing conservatorship." I have used names that are either common or self-explanatory, but you may encounter different terms, laws, and regulations in your own state or county.

Your case will be shaped by the specific facts of your situation and by the particular laws of your state. If you need legal advice, talk to an attorney who specializes in your specific area of law: family law, guardianship, juvenile dependency, and so on. He or she can advise you on the basis of the facts and circumstances of your individual case and the laws that apply in your state.

YOUR RIGHTS AS A GRANDPARENT

"Grandparents have all the responsibilities and none of the rights," says one grandmother.[2] "The courts treat you as though you're some old busybody who just doesn't like the way your kids are raising their kids," complains another. "They act as though you have no right whatsoever to care about these babies."[3]

It's not an uncommon feeling among relatives caught up in the legal system. One of the reasons is that while families and courts may share similar goals—in most cases, the best interest of the child in question— they come to those goals from different places. Grandparents and other relatives have a heart connection to the child; their actions and goals are driven by love. The court is a legal authority in regard to the child; its actions and goals are driven by laws, rules, and regulations. When these two groups are thrown together around emotionally charged issues of family and resources, the dynamic can be challenging—more so for relatives, since the final decision-making authority often rests with the court.

However, grandparents don't always understand the rights and responsibilities they do have or how those rights interact with the rights of the parents and the rights of the child.

Every family member has the right to care *about* a child, but the right to take care *of* a child who is not your own is a legal right, that is, conferred by law. According to attorney Joseph MacKenzie, "Too often, caregivers don't ask about their legal rights and wait too long to assert their legal interests in a child: after an unstable parent suddenly shows up and takes the child away from the only home he has known, or after child protective services takes the child because someone called the child abuse hotline to report that the child was abused, neglected, or abandoned by the parents."[4]

Historically, American parents have had almost exclusive authority over their children. Our government cannot dictate how people raise their families, nor can it randomly take their children away from them. There are countries where the government can easily interfere with family relationships. Just imagine a social worker, lawyer, or relative being able to come into your house to tell you how to raise your own kids, and you may see why parental rights are important. Unless a child is in some kind of danger—seriously neglected, abandoned, or at significant risk of injury or harm—no one, not even the court, can interfere with the parent–child relationship. Even when a child is legally removed from a parent's care, every effort is made to enable him to return safely home.

Grandparenthood, in our society, is a biological connection, not necessarily a legal one. The grandparent–grandchild relationship can be legally severed by adoption, divorce, and even the whim of an angry parent. (Although even the parent–child relationship can be legally severed if a child's continued safety is at risk.)

But it is the rights of the child that are central to most legal proceedings regarding custody and visitation, and that includes a child's right to a safe and stable relationship with his parents whenever possible.

There was a time when children's rights were not recognized. Basically, they were treated as property. Parents could put their children to work and punish them in any way they saw fit. Today we recognize— and support with legislation and case law—the rights of children, which include the right to be free from abuse and neglect, to have a relationship with both parents (assuming the child is safe), and, more recently, to have court-appointed legal representation in juvenile court dependency proceedings. We have institutions and systems in place to protect the welfare of children, and "the best interests of the child" is the legal standard commonly used in custody and visitation cases. There is no simple or single legal definition of "best interest," however. The guidelines are intentionally broad so that the court can consider individual situations, circumstances, and relationships in determining what's best for each child.

So do you, as a grandparent, have legal rights? You do. But they are much more limited than the rights you had as a parent. You have a right to *file* for the guardianship of a child in your family or in your care. If a child is removed from parental custody, federal law grants grandparents and other relatives the right to be *considered* for custody and the right to request *de facto* parent status in dependency court proceedings. And in most states, grandparents have the right to *petition* for visitation. None of these outcomes is guaranteed, but the right to request them in court represents a legal recognition of the importance of extended family. These rights, however, still relate more to government policy regarding the interests of the child than to your inherent rights as a grandparent or relative.

Once you become an active relative caregiver for a child, other rights and responsibilities come into play (more on this below and in Chapter 11). In the end, however, it is the child whose rights are most rigorously represented in a court of law. "Grandparents often think it's the parent," says MacKenzie. "But it's really about the children and their relationships with the adults who parent them. Parents have a constitutional right to their children, and children have a right to their parents." In other words, grandparent issues come under your grandchild's right to a relationship with *you.* "You can call it grandparent's rights," he adds, "but it's really a matter of children's rights. That's why they're called 'dependents'; they have to depend on others to take good care of them."[5]

This is an important distinction to keep in mind as you approach the legal system on your grandchild's behalf. The more you can align your actions and your explanations with the guiding principle of the court, that is, "the best interests of the child," the better chance you have of affecting a positive outcome for everyone involved.

THE LEGAL CUSTODY OF GRANDCHILDREN

Lack of legal custody is one of the main issues facing grandparents who are raising grandchildren in their homes. Without legal custody, you may have problems enrolling a child in school, putting a child on your medical insurance policy, getting him medical care, or seeking government aid. Without legal custody, you have no control over whether your grandchild is handed back to an abusive, neglectful, or intoxicated parent. Even with some kind of custody arrangement, your power to make parental decisions for your grandchild may be limited.

Custody defines a relationship of control over and responsibility for a minor child. The word *custody* is confusing because people use that word to mean many different things. A grandfather whose grandson lives with him may say that he has "custody" of his grandson. A grandmother whose granddaughters were placed with her by the court may call that "custody." Grandparents who have legal guardianship of their grandchild will say they have "custody." And each does have a small piece of the custody puzzle.

Basically, there are two kinds of custody—physical and legal—and that is where the confusion lies. If a child lives with you, she is in your *physical* custody, but you may not necessarily have *legal* custody. Physical custody means physical care of and control over a child, including the right to have her live with you. Legal custody means legal authority to make decisions about the medical, educational, health, and welfare needs of the child. These distinctions are common in divorce and child custody settlements, where both parents may have "joint custody" (shared legal and physical responsibility for a child) or one parent may have sole legal and physical custody, while the other parent may have visitation rights. But divorce is not the only circumstance that puts the custody of a child in question. The legal system can transfer the custody of a child in order to protect her from danger. This is where grandparents come into the picture.

If your grandchild lives with you, the child is physically in your custody, whether you have an informal arrangement or a formal one. The more critical questions are these: Who has legal custody? What is your legal relationship to the grandchild in your care? What are your legal rights, duties, and responsibilities as the child's caregiver? And what are the limitations of your arrangement?

There are four types of custody situations that may affect your grandchild: informal custody, court placement (and/or foster care), guardianship, and adoption. Each has legal and financial consequences for your family. Another issue you may be involved with as a grandparent is visitation. While this is not a matter of custody, it affects many grandparents deeply.

Informal Custody

Many grandparents who have grandchildren living with them have no legal arrangements for doing so. They start out caring for the children on a casual basis and seem to continue that way. Some grandparents don't even realize that there are legal options available to them. This makes informal custody one of the most common arrangements among grandparents. With informal custody you have, in essence, physical custody of the child while legal custody remains with the parents. Unfortunately, this situation offers the least protection for you and your grandchildren because there is no court order to enforce the arrangement.

Informal custody can mean constant struggles over school enrollment, medical care, and financial assistance. Many school districts may not allow a nonparent to enroll a child in school unless he is the legal guardian. Relatives also can run into difficulties obtaining medical care for a minor child.

On the plus side, informal custody means you don't have high court costs and attorney fees, and you don't have government involvement with your family. But it also means that you are at the mercy of the child's parents; they can take the child whenever they want to, and you will have no legal means to stop them. You are, in fact, little more than a glorified baby-sitter. If you only have informal custody of your grandchildren, you have no real control over their safety. As long as you are without legal protection, you are open to parental manipulation.

■ HOW TO COPE

• *Look into government aid.* Just because you have informal custody of your grandchildren does not mean you must shoulder the financial burden alone. Your grandchildren may be entitled to financial and medical assistance through one of several government programs (see Chapter 12 for details).

• *Look into guardianship.* If your grandchildren are not in the custody of the juvenile dependency system, you may be able to file for guardianship. Not only is this the most stable arrangement for your grandchildren (short of adoption), but if you apply for guardianship early enough, it can keep you out of the juvenile courts and prevent interference from child protective services. If your grandchildren's safety is not at risk, and you do not need to involve the police or child protective services, consider private guardianship (see "Guardianship," below).

• *Consider a power of attorney.* Power of attorney gives one person the legal right to make decisions for another. For instance, a single mother could give someone power of attorney to enroll a child in school or give emergency medical consent if she is out of town. In doing so, the mother doesn't give up any parental rights; she only allows another person to make certain decisions. Power of attorney can be a useful temporary solution when a parent is incarcerated and wants a relative to care for a child or when a parent travels extensively. Of course, a document like this is only useful if officials choose to accept it, and it can always be rescinded by the parents. If you are in a situation that does not require or allow for guardianship, at least ask the parents for power of attorney.

• *Consider a Relative Caregiver Affidavit.* Some states allow relative caregivers to fill out a legal document that allows them to enroll a child in school and consent to medical care. A Relative Caregiver Affidavit (sometimes called a Caregiver's Authorization Affidavit) does not take away or suspend parental rights and must typically be renewed after a year, but it does make it easier for you to interact with schools and doctors if you don't have legal custody or a Power of Attorney. If your grandchild stops living with you, you should immediately notify the school and any other agency that was given a copy of the affidavit.

Court Placement and Foster Care

Foster care provides temporary substitute parenting to children whose parents can not or will not take care of them. It is part of an emergency response system that is designed to protect children who are suspected of being abused or neglected or who have been abandoned. Foster care usually starts with a call to a social worker, the police, or a child abuse hotline. The children may then be taken into protective custody while the juvenile dependency system decides whether or not to remove them from their parents and make them "dependents of the court." When a child becomes a dependent of the court, the judge, the social worker, and the child's attorney all share responsibility for tracking the child's well-being. This includes such issues as placement, family visitation, health care, dental and mental health services, and the child's educational needs.

Custody of your grandchild changes when she becomes a dependent of the court. The court retains legal custody of the child, but someone is awarded physical custody. That someone has traditionally been a foster parent. Foster parents are appointed to care for a child while the court conducts a series of hearings to determine if the allegations against the parents are true and, if so, how to protect the child. These hearings are generally called "dependency hearings."

Most people associate foster care with care by strangers. However, because of increasing numbers of children needing court protection and a growing acknowledgment of the importance of family bonds to healthy child development, states have begun to rely increasingly on relatives. This makes court placement the most common *legal* arrangement for grandparents.

With court placement, grandparents have a limited degree of custody. You have physical custody of the child (that is, he lives with you) and limited authority to enroll him in school and seek medical attention, but the court and child welfare agency retain legal custody. Court placement gives you more legal protection than does an informal custody arrangement—and the possibility of higher government benefits—but you also have a kind of marriage to the system. You will be expected to comply with court visitation, to encourage "reunification" with the parents, and to submit your family to the scrutiny of the local child welfare agency. You exchange the possibility of parental interference for the certainty of interference by social workers, attorneys, and judges (and generally without any choice in the matter).

There are differences between court placement with a relative and foster care, mainly in terms of licensing requirements and government assistance. Foster parents must be trained and licensed to have children in their homes. They may be licensed only for a fixed number of children, for certain ages, and sometimes for one sex. They must also supply separate bedrooms for girls and boys and one bed per child. Many states also limit the number of children per room. Relatives must also be approved by social services before a child can be placed with them—a process that includes a home inspection and background checks for you and all the adults in your home—but they don't usually have to go through the training and licensing process.

The other difference between court placement with a relative and foster care involves financial aid. Federal funds may be available to support children who are in the custody of the state, and these benefits are significantly higher than welfare benefits. Some states also provide their own programs for children who don't qualify for federal foster care. Children placed with relatives are also entitled to government support. (See Chapter 12 for more information on government aid.)

If you have a grandchild in the dependency system, the individual laws of your state will determine if he is placed in your custody and under what conditions. The best thing you can do is educate yourself about the dependency process and try to comply with your state regulations. (See Chapter 11 for a discussion of child protective services and the dependency system.)

Guardianship

Outside of adoption, legal guardianship is the safest, most stable arrangement for a grandparent raising a grandchild. In fact, legal guardianship *is* custody, both physical and legal. It is the legal transfer of custody to someone other than a parent. This can happen with parental consent or when one or both of the parents are dead, missing, or unfit. The first two categories are straightforward; "unfit" is a murkier concept. Nevertheless, unfit parents have become a common cause of guardianship actions. As attorney Teresa de la O told the Santa Rosa *Press Democrat,* "We've always done them [guardianships], but it used to be when one parent died and the other wasn't all that interested in having the child. Now we're doing it because neither parent is parenting."[6]

Legal guardianship does not terminate parental rights, but it does suspend them. It is a formal agreement that must be granted by a court and signed by a judge. With guardianship, you acquire rights and responsibilities that are similar, if not equal, to those of a parent. As attorney Harold LaFlamme puts it: "You step into the shoes of the parent. You don't have a pink slip, but something close."[7]

The advantage of guardianship is control. You decide where your grandchild lives (within the state). You have legal authority to enroll her in school, consent to general medical treatment, and make many of the decisions a parent can make in terms of education, sports, health care, employment, and legal actions. You must provide for the safety, protection, and physical and emotional growth of the child. You also have control over when and how your grandchild sees her parents, unless there is a court-ordered visitation schedule. The parent may retain some rights, similar to joint custody in a divorce settlement, but you have legal control. And you are not at the beck and call of the dependency court.

What you cannot do as a guardian is make decisions about the child's religion or move the child out of state without the court's permission. Although you are not entitled to any of the child's earnings or property, you are responsible for the care and safety of the child and for any damage she does while you are guardian.

The disadvantages of applying for legal guardianship are the cost and the risk to relationships. Filing for private guardianship can mean high attorney fees and court costs, particularly if the parents or other relatives contest your petition.

There are also emotional risks in filing for guardianship. Unless the parents have died or disappeared, you are petitioning to suspend parental rights. This requires proving that the parent is unfit and detrimental to the child. You will have to build a case against the parent that involves more than the separation anxiety your grandchild will suffer if he is removed from your home. You will have to show things like a history of irresponsibility, drug abuse, physical or sexual abuse, or a lack of residence, as well as the effect such factors will have on the child. You will also have to prove that it is in the child's best interests to be with you. You will not endear yourself to your adult child by painting these pictures and taking custody of the child. If you win, you guarantee some security for your grandchild. But, warns attorney LaFlamme, "If you lose, you could lose big: the money and the relationship with your child and grandchild."[8]

Even at its best, guardianship is never permanent. Under normal circumstances, it lasts until the child is 18, marries, becomes emancipated (recognized as an adult), or is adopted.[9] However, you can be removed as a guardian by the court at any time if it is proven that returning your grandchild to the parents or assigning another guardian is in the child's best interests. Only adoption offers airtight custody.

Filing for Guardianship

To file for private guardianship, you or your attorney must file several legal forms, often called a "guardianship petition," in whichever branch of your civil court handles guardianship (generally either probate, juvenile, or family law). You must also notify in writing *all* the child's parents and grandparents, maternal and paternal. These family members will be notified of all hearings and given an opportunity to object to your petition and to seek custody for themselves. You will also have to pay filing and investigation fees, the cost of which can vary.

If there is an emergency situation or you believe the child is at immediate risk and in need of protection, you can often ask the court to grant you "temporary guardianship" until the hearing. This is one way to keep the children safe with you while you file for custody.

Once a hearing date is set, a state or county agency will conduct an investigation to decide if the guardianship is necessary. In most states the social service agency will also run a background check on you for any arrests or involvement with child protective services. The agency may also conduct an investigation of your home and may interview your grandchild if she is old enough. At the guardianship hearing, the judge will consider the petition, the social service investigator's report, and all the available testimony before making a final decision.

If there is no opposition to your petition from parents or other relatives, seeking guardianship can be a relatively simple procedure. If, however, the parents or other relatives contest your guardianship petition, they can hire their own attorneys and confront you in a full hearing. This is where the cost of court and attorney fees can start to climb.

Guardianship through Dependency

It is possible to obtain guardianship through the dependency system but only at the final stages of the dependency process. If by the final hearing (called the "permanency hearing") the judge decides that the child cannot safely return home, he or she will order adoption, guardianship, or another planned permanency living arrangement (formerly called "long-term foster care") as the best plan for the child. If guardianship is granted, the court may close the child's dependency case. (For more on the dependency process, see Chapter 11. See also "Foster Care Assistance" in Chapter 12.)

Standby and Short-Term Guardianship

A "standby guardianship" is a guardianship order issued with the parent's consent for some point in the future. For instance, if a single mother has cancer, she can set up a standby guardianship that takes effect upon her death (as long as there is no other parent to object and the court doesn't find it harmful to the child). Short-term guardianship is just that: a legal custody arrangement for a limited period of time and with a predetermined termination date. For instance, Illinois parents can appoint a short-term guardian for up to 365 days without a court order.[10] This allows incarcerated parents to provide legal care for their children while they serve time and still regain custody upon their release.

If you are caring for a child whose parents are sick or in jail, find out if your state offers standby or short-term guardianship arrangements.

■ WHAT YOU NEED TO KNOW

• *Sometimes court costs can be waived.* In some states you can apply for a waiver of court fees and costs if you can show financial hardship. The application is sometimes called a pauper's waiver or *in forma pauperis* application. If you currently receive financial assistance for yourself (not your grandchild) in the form of disability or welfare benefits, food stamps, or any other form of general relief, you may qualify for this waiver.

• *You may be able to "do it yourself."* Some states make it possible to apply for guardianship without an attorney, particularly if the guardianship petition is uncontested. There may be books, manuals, and websites that explain the process in your state. If you don't need or cannot afford an attorney, find out if you can apply for guardianship without one. Contact your local Legal Aid office for information.

• *You must prove that it is harmful to the child to continue in the parent's custody.* Just because you are currently raising your grandchild is not enough reason for a judge to make you a guardian. Parents have a right to ask someone else to care for a child, particularly when they are in and out of the picture, without it being considered abandonment. If, on the other hand, the parent has disappeared for a significant amount of time, you may have a better chance for guardianship to be granted.

• *You must also show that the child is better off with you.* Be careful when you do this; reasons like better income can backfire. The court is not going to give you your grandchildren just because you can provide more for them economically. Unless they are being abused or neglected, a judge is unlikely to interfere. As an attorney once told me, "We don't want to take custody away from poor people just because they're poor." What kind of information is the court looking for? Information about the physical and emotional health of the child; how the child behaves after visits with the parent; proof of your ability to provide a stable home environment if the parents cannot.

• *Parents will often be granted visitation rights.* A parent who doesn't have custody is entitled to reasonable visitation in a guardianship situation, unless the court decides that visitation poses a danger to the child's physical, mental, or emotional health. Even jailed parents may be granted visits if the court believes that they are in the best interests of the child. If either parent is granted visitation, be prepared to cooperate.

• *You can protect your grandchildren.* As a legal guardian you can determine where and when an unstable parent sees your grandchild. You can even get a "Stay Away" order or a restraining order, if necessary. But you must be able to show the court that the parent is a threat to you or to your grandchild's safety. Many grandparents won't get restraining orders against their adult children for fear of retaliation. It can also be difficult to call the police on your own son or daughter. But if you do have to call the police, a restraining order gives you more credibility.

• *Guardianship is always temporary.* Even if your grandchild has lived with you since birth, the court can revoke your guardianship status. However, while parents can file a petition and request the court to overturn a guardianship arrangement, they must prove that they can safely care for the child and that this change in custody is in the child's best interest. This is rarely accomplished when the problem is substance abuse.

Pam and Robert Marshall clearly understand this. They filed for custody of their granddaughter when the drug-addicted mother, Linda, was in jail (the father is unknown). "I know that guardianship can be overturned," says Pam, "but what it does is temporarily protect Megan. Linda would have to go into court and prove she has a home, a job, stability, and could take care of her. As of yesterday, I doubt that."

- *Don't give up.* People will tell you many things. For instance, several attorneys told Pam Marshall that no court would allow her to take custody of a granddaughter. While your state laws may prevent you from filing for guardianship, don't just take anyone's word for it. "No matter what anyone tells you, do it anyway," says one grandmother. "I was told I could not win. And you know what? I have three healthy, happy grandchildren."

- *Protect your paperwork.* Your guardianship documents are the proof that you are your grandchild's legal guardian. Keep them in a safe place.

Adoption

In many states you can adopt your own grandchildren under certain circumstances: for example, when the child is orphaned or legally abandoned, when the parents consent to the adoption, or when their parental rights are terminated by trial or the dependency court system.

Adoption is the most secure custody arrangement available to nonparents. It permanently dissolves all legal ties between parent and child and creates a new parent–child relationship in the eyes of the law. In effect, you would no longer be grandparents to your grandchild but new parents, with all the rights and responsibilities of biological parents. To quote one child welfare agency, "When you adopt a child, your legal relationship with that child is the same as with a child born to you."[11]

Adoption gives you full legal custody. It means the end of continual court appearances, and it means that the parent can never again contest or interfere. As an adoptive parent you can now move your grandchild out of state, if you choose, and allow her to inherit directly from you. You also acquire the full legal and financial responsibility for parenting the child. Unlike guardianship, adoption means that your relationship is permanent, extending past the child's 18th birthday, just as with your own children.

Adoption also means peace of mind, not only for you but for your grandchildren, who don't have to worry about ever being taken away again. Nancy Harper's granddaughter Marissa was thrilled when her grandmother adopted her. She thought it was wonderful that the judge said that she could stay with Grandma for the rest of her life and never leave. I heard about a little boy who took his stuffed bear to court with him. When the judge asked about it, he replied, "Well, he's always been at my Grandma's too, and he wants to know if he can be adopted, too, because he never wants to leave Grandma's house, either." Today, both boy and bear are legally adopted.

If adoption is such an airtight solution to the custody nightmares, you might ask, "Why don't more grandparents pursue it?" There are several reasons.

• *Grandparents don't easily give up on their adult children, and adoption means terminating the rights of the parent.* It can be a difficult emotional choice to make. On one hand, adopting a grandchild is a relief: It validates the fact that you are raising your grandchild and ends your dealings with social workers and the courts. On the other hand, it means admitting defeat where your adult child is concerned. Says attorney Robert Walmsley, "In terms of the grandparents, adoption is generally the last resort, when they see no hope of the adult child ever being responsible. Parenthood is precious. You hoped your child would shape up. By this point, you've lost all hope."[12]

• *Many grandparents believe that adoption is unnecessary because they and the children are already family.* They may also hesitate to adopt because the parents are still in the picture. The fact that the birth parents may continue to interact with the children can make grandparent adoption confusing and complicated. Because ties are not severed, children may be confused about whom to listen to and may be prevented from making a clean start with Grandma and Grandpa as a new family.

• *It is difficult to terminate a parent's rights.* Unless the parents consent to the adoption, have already lost custody, or are completely out of the picture, you may need to prove that your own child is unfit to raise his or her own children. This can involve a full trial with witnesses; everything about your family will be open to scrutiny.

• *Adoption is costly.* Not only do you have court costs, but unless your grandchildren are eligible for adoption assistance, you can also lose access to government aid. Many grandparents don't adopt their grandchildren because they live on a fixed income and can't afford to raise children without welfare benefits. However, the adoption tax credit might help you recoup out-of-pocket expenses. Ask a tax consultant about current eligibility and documentation requirements, or check the resources at the North American Council on Adoptable Children (NACAC). (See Appendix A for contact information.)

• *Your age can become a negative factor if the adoption is contested.* One New Hampshire couple had legal guardianship of their son's two children for two years before filing for adoption. Fourteen months into the trial, a young couple on the mother's side contested the adoption and won.

If you are considering adopting your grandchild, here are some things you might want to consider:

- You will be a full legal parent again. Are you ready for that?
- Will the parents continue to interact with the child? How will you handle that?
- Does the child have a relationship with the parents? How will adoption affect that relationship?
- How old is the child and how does he or she feel about the adoption? After a certain age—10 to 14, depending on the state[13]—children have the right to consent to an adoption.
- How is your health? Do you have the stamina and good health to commit to raising another set of children?
- What is your financial situation? If you are getting government aid, can you afford to give it up? Are you eligible for adoption assistance? (See Chapter 12.)

If you decide to go ahead with the adoption, consult a good adoption attorney—as well as a therapist about the impact this move could have on your grandchild and your family. If the child is old enough, listen closely to what he or she has to say about it. Some children are eager to cut their ties to their parents, others will object.

VISITATION

Legal visitation is not a form of custody, but it is an important issue when the custody of a child changes. In a divorce, for instance, the mother may get legal custody and the father may receive visitation privileges. The grandparents can sometimes be left out in the cold. However, divorce is not the only situation in which grandparents are prevented from seeing their grandchildren. Grandparents may also be denied visitation in the following circumstances:

- A daughter dies and the husband remarries.
- An unmarried son fathers a child and the mother moves away.
- A stepparent adopts the grandchildren.
- A grandchild is placed in foster care.
- A married daughter simply refuses to let her parents see their grandchildren.

Even grandparents who have raised a child for years can lose total access to that child if the parents reappear or regain custody. One Ohio grandmother provided day care for her married daughter for 50 hours a week for four years; after a family argument, the parents refused her even occasional visitation. In situations like these, many grandparents turn to the law for help.

Grandparent Visitation and State Laws

Almost every state in the United States has some kind of grandparent visitation statute. These statutes do not give grandparents a legal right to visit a grandchild but a right to *petition* for visitation. The court reserves the right to refuse any petition based on the merits of the case. Each statute defines who may petition for visitation, when, and under what circumstances. Some states also outline what standard the court should apply in awarding visitation, usually "the best interests of the child."

- *Who may petition.* While most states only allow grandparents to petition for visitation, some states extend the privilege to great-grandparents, siblings, and other relatives.
- *When you may petition.* Many states limit the right to petition to specific circumstances, such as the divorce or death of a parent. However, some states include additional circumstances, such as incarcera-

tion of the parent; abandonment of the child; when the child is born out of wedlock; and when custody has been given to a third party or when the child has been placed in foster care. Others even allow grandparents to seek visitation when the parents are still married. Although adoption usually cuts all ties between a child and his or her biological family, some states allow grandparents to petition for visitation in instances when a grandchild has been adopted by a stepparent or other relative.

Visitation in Dependency

If a child is removed from the parents by child protective services and is not placed with you, the court may consider whether it is in his best interests to have visits with you. Many factors can influence this decision, including your prior relationship with the child and whether such visitation might interfere with parental reunification.

If the parents' rights are terminated by the court, your relationship with your grandchild could terminate as well. Some states do allow grandparents to petition for visitation when a child is adopted by a stepparent or relative but not when the adoptive parents are unrelated.

■ HOW TO COPE

• *Know the law.* Visitation laws vary. Find out the parameters of your own state's visitation laws and proceed accordingly.

• *Consider alternatives to legal action.* Litigation is not only expensive but also time-consuming, and it can permanently damage already fragile family relationships. Once a lawsuit starts, people cling to their own side of the story and stop listening. Animosity grows. The children are the ones who get caught in the cross fire. Furthermore, while people's feelings constantly change and evolve, court decisions are fixed and inflexible. Is there anything you can do to keep your family out of the courtroom? Would family counseling address the parent's unwillingness to allow visitation? Is mediation a possibility? Some states have informal dispute resolution or mediation services to help settle visitation problems. If you must battle in court to see your grandchild, it can certainly be worth the fight, but first try to seek other alternatives.

WHEN YOU NEED AN ATTORNEY

At some point in this second parenthood you may need to consult an attorney. Perhaps your grandchild has ended up as a dependent of the court and you risk losing her to the system. Perhaps you are trying for guardianship. Maybe you don't have your grandchild, but you are petitioning for visitation rights. Each of these can be an overwhelming legal struggle, and you may want an expert on your side. Even if you are settled in a comfortable custody situation, there are other battles to fight on behalf of your grandchild—with various agencies for proper government aid; with your school district for proper educational services; even with hospitals and Medicaid for medical coverage. Although you are your grandchild's best advocate, sometimes even the sharpest advocate needs help.

Do You Need Legal Counsel?

Whether or not you need an attorney depends on what it is you are trying to accomplish. If everything is going smoothly or you are filing an uncontested visitation and guardianship agreement, you may not need an attorney. Much will depend on the laws of your state.

On the other hand, you do want to hire an attorney whenever the parent or parents hire one first; it keeps the playing field level. You may also need an attorney if you are contesting a judicial proceeding, petitioning to become part of a proceeding, filing a contested visitation or guardianship petition, adopting a child, or appealing an administrative decision.

If you have a question you can't answer, you may need to consult with an attorney, but you may not need to hire one to represent you. Consultation fees vary. Each state has its own laws about when you can and cannot legally represent yourself, but one thing is certain: If you feel you need an attorney, you should consider hiring one.

What to Look For

Attorneys, like doctors, have different specialties. If you petition for guardianship, you don't want an attorney who specializes in divorce or dependency. And if a dependency hearing is imminent, you need an attorney who really knows that system. In other words, know what you're looking for, and do your research.

When you look for legal counsel, you also want to make sure your case is not the first grandparent case your attorney has handled. This is where knowledge is power. Learn the terms. Then make sure your attorney knows them. Does he understand the ins and outs of the dependency process? Can he discuss changes in visitation law? If not, find someone who can.

It is just as important to make sure your attorney believes in your case. When a South Carolina couple wanted to mount a legal battle for their grandson, they were discouraged by an attorney who told them, "He's got parents."[14] This is not an attorney you want working for you.

Where to Look

Where you look for an attorney or an advocate depends on your resources and circumstances. Attorneys charge by the hour, and their rates vary according to your location, the size of their firm, and the difficulty of the case. Your total cost will also depend on what needs to be accomplished; filing a document will cost considerably less than a protracted fight in court. One grandmother's attorney told her that her custody battle with the child's mother would cost her "a room addition and a trip to Europe" before they were finished, and he wasn't far off. On the other hand, some cases can be simple and straightforward.

Your best source for legal referrals is other grandparents and grandparent support groups. Which attorneys have other people worked with? What were their experiences? They know which ones are effective and which ones are not. Also, if you are involved in a dependency case, you might consider asking the court clerks which lawyers they recommend.

If you are on a fixed income, you will have a smaller pool to choose from, but you still have options. Ask your state or local bar association if any family law attorneys work "pro bono" (that is, donate legal assistance) or at reduced rates. Contact your local Legal Aid organization or legal services office to find out about free or low-cost representation for people who are income eligible. A law school or law clinic might even provide free voluntary services to people on fixed or limited incomes.

Court-Appointed Attorneys

Many states offer court-appointed attorneys to key parties in a dependency case who cannot afford their own attorneys, namely, parents who have been accused of abusing or neglecting their children and, sometimes, the children themselves. A court-appointed attorney has the same obligations as a private attorney in terms of representing her clients in court. Occasionally, a grandparent or relative will be eligible for a court-appointed attorney. Some states allow relatives and foster parents who have acted as day-to-day parents in a child's life to petition for "de facto parent" status and become a party in a case, which gives them the right to be present at court procedures and to provide evidence and cross-examine witnesses. If these de facto parents cannot afford an attorney, in some jurisdictions, the court may appoint one for them (although it is not required to do so).

While a court-appointed attorney can be a financial help, this method of acquiring legal counsel can be a game of Russian roulette in terms of an attorney's sensitivity. You could get a compassionate, caring individual who truly supports your case or one of those who are just doing their job. One grandmother's court-appointed attorney, speaking to me on behalf of her client, told me she was "dumb as dirt" and "too emotional." The risk is even greater when the only attorney in the picture is a court-appointed attorney for the child. In this case, he is only bound to represent the child. Whether or not your view is ever heard will depend on the attorney and how sympathetic that individual is to grandparents.

If your court-appointed attorney is wonderful, treasure her. Unfortunately, there isn't much you can do if you're unhappy with your attorney. You can request a replacement, but you may not get one.

■ HOW TO COPE

• *Be persistent.* If your attorney doesn't return your calls in a timely fashion, keep calling back. Attorneys have busy schedules and busy office staffs; sometimes messages fall through the cracks.

• *Tell your attorney the whole truth.* Tell the negative as well as the positive. Don't hide anything. Withholding information because you fear it could hurt your case can do more damage than telling the truth. If you have something in your past that could cause trouble—for instance, a jail record from your youth—let your attorney know. He can address the problem in a way that could minimize damage to your case. If you don't tell him, and the other side finds out, they could have a field day in court. So tell him everything you can think of, even if it doesn't seem important. Your attorney is the best judge of which facts can harm, or help, your case.

11

Child Protection and the Dependency System

> You have to have an understanding of what the dependency law is, for a grandparent, to understand what kind of Pandora's box you are opening when you make that one call to CPS [child protective services].
>
> —*Ted Youmans, attorney*[1]

Claire and Evan Powers basically raised their granddaughter, Sarah, until she was 10 years old. Sarah had arrived in the world with the deck stacked against her: a father who drank, a mother on drugs, and an abusive relationship between the two. Claire and Evan, her paternal grandparents, were her ace in the hole. They often let her mother stay the night or agreed to keep baby Sarah with them when violence broke out at home. Almost from the beginning, Sarah was in and out of Grandma's house.

Then, when Sarah was 18 months old, her parents split up. Dad wanted the baby off the streets, so Mom and Sarah moved in with Evan and Claire. After a few months Mom took Sarah and disappeared without warning. When Dad found them in a crack house six months later, he sued for custody. While the case was still pending, Mom showed up with Sarah. "I can't take care of her anymore," she told Claire. "I'll be back in three months." Then Mom took off without the baby. Dad got custody of two-year-old Sarah, but Grandma and Grandpa got the bulk of the responsibility. Over the next four years they bought her clothes, took her to the day care center, and baby-sat, sometimes for a week at a time. Sarah was spending more and more time at Grandma's house, until eventually father and daughter moved in with Evan and Claire.

By this time, however, Dad was also using drugs and was increasingly abusive to his parents and his daughter. He eventually left and moved into a motel near a crack house. One day he decided he didn't want his parents to have Sarah anymore; he packed her up and took her down to the crack house with him. Claire called the sheriff. She had previously called child abuse hotlines three times due to her son's drug use and abuse of Sarah, but each time she was told there was not enough evidence. This time, when she called, they acted. Sarah's father was arrested at the crack house; Sarah was taken into protective custody and placed back with Claire. Finally, Claire thought, her problems were over. Little did she know they were just beginning.

When Claire called the sheriff, she started the wheels of justice turning. The wheels of justice, she discovered, can sometimes run over the very people they are meant to help. The social services agency not only started dependency court proceedings against Dad but went out looking for Mom, who had not been seen for several years.

Sarah's mother had been a heavy drug user for most of Sarah's life. She knew where to find her daughter, but she had never contacted her, sent letters, or offered support. She had no parental relationship with the child. In fact, Sarah barely knew her mother, who was living on the streets when she was located. Still, the legal system provided Mom with a free lawyer, reunification services, a drug rehabilitation program, and, eventually, Sarah. All of this was done despite the facts that Mom had essentially abandoned the child, that she had been investigated for child abuse three times before Sarah was six months old, and most importantly, that Sarah told everyone—the social worker, the judge, her own attorney, her grandparents, and her mother—that she didn't want to go with her mother, that the only home she had known was with Grandma and Grandpa. "Sarah jumped up on my lap in court and hugged me; I was crying," Claire recalls. "She thought she was going home with me because she had told the judge that she wanted to." But that is not what the judge ordered.

Today Sarah is 12 years old and living with her mother. She has lost weight, has trouble sleeping, and has developed behavioral problems. Claire and Evan are permitted to see her for only one weekend each month, and achieving that right cost them $35,000 in legal fees. Mom doesn't make it easy, either: Visits are never hassle free, and Mom sends Sarah to her grandparents for three days with only the clothes on her back. "She would like people to believe she's clean, but I don't think she is," says Claire. "Even the judge said, at the time, that the mother has unresolved drug problems and the boyfriend is an alcoholic, but the judge had to protect the mother's custodial rights. These were rights she'd had for years and never used."

Claire and Evan Powers lost their granddaughter by calling a system they thought would help them. Claire says that call was her "biggest mistake ever." In her eyes, the system protects the parents. It gives them attorneys, and it gives them services. "They follow them around with a pillow so if they fall down they don't get bruised," she says bitterly.

Looked at another way, however, Claire and Evan lost Sarah because they weren't aware of their legal rights or options. They had no understanding of the legal system and didn't know how to protect their granddaughter or their relationship with her. They waited until it was too late to secure legal rights and to establish a legal relationship. They didn't know it could be done, and they didn't know how to do it. To quote one attorney, "Just as childhood does not wait for parents to get their lives together, the law does not wait when children get caught up in the legal system."[2]

"The system." Grandparents shudder when they talk about it. These two words seem to stand for everything impersonal, overbearing, and bureaucratic in government, for power gone out of control. When grandparents talk about "the system," they mean the dependency system (also called the child welfare system). It is the combination of child protection agencies and juvenile court proceedings designed to protect and aid children in crisis.

Many grandparents have never dealt with the system before because they raised their own children without interference from courts and social workers. Even those who are familiar with the system find that involvement as a grandparent is completely different from involvement as a parent. In any case, the dependency process can be an overwhelming and frustrating experience. All grandparents need to know about this process—not only for protection if they find themselves in the system, but to learn when, how, and why to avoid it.

WHAT IS THE DEPENDENCY SYSTEM?

The dependency system is part of the government's emergency response to protect minor children who are suspected of being abused, neglected, or abandoned. Every state has at least one part of its child welfare agency dedicated to investigating reports of children in crisis—often called child protective services (CPS)—and at least one court, typically the juvenile court, responsible for deciding these cases.

The dependency process is a series of hearings in which a judge decides whether allegations against the parents* are true and, if so, how to protect the child while the parents try to solve their problems. Among the issues considered in the various dependency hearings are the following:

- Whether the child should be removed from the home.
- Where the child should be placed during the dependency process.
- What measures, such as drug rehabilitation and counseling, the parents must take to regain custody of the child.
- What the court can do to help the parents reunite with the child (for example, devise a visitation schedule or order parenting classes).
- What services, such as counseling, the court can recommend for the child.
- How the family is progressing.
- If and when the child can safely return home.
- What permanent custody arrangement can be made if the child cannot return home (permanent plans are generally a choice of adoption, guardianship, or long-term foster care, which is now referred to as "another planned permanent living arrangement").

During the course of these hearings the child is considered a "dependent of the court" (thus the term "dependency hearings"). This means that

---

*For simplicity, we are using the plural "parents" throughout this discussion. It is understood that in many cases only one parent may be involved.

legal custody of the child transfers from the parents to the state (whereas physical custody will be awarded to someone who can care for the child). The dependency system is, for many children, a doorway into foster care; however, federal law gives preference to placing children with relatives rather than in foster homes whenever possible and appropriate.

The Goals of Dependency

The primary goal of the dependency system is to make sure that children are safe and free from abuse, even if that means removing them from their parents' care. If a child must be removed from his parents' custody, the next goal is "family reunification," to help the parents solve their problems so that the child can return safely home. Toward that end, the system will offer parents services like therapy, drug and alcohol treatment, domestic violence programs, parenting classes, anything to help them correct the problems that led to their losing custody and to help them reunify with their children. If reunification is not possible—and only once that is clear—then the final goal is to find a safe and permanent living situation for the child.

Federal law supports placing children with relatives, both as an alternative to foster care and, if it eventually becomes necessary, as a permanent plan through adoption or kinship guardianship. However, if a child is placed with you, as a relative caregiver, you must actively encourage the parent–child relationship. The court will place a child with strangers rather than let family members interfere with reunification. This can be devastating, particularly if you are prevented from seeing or contacting your grandchild as a result.

The Power of Dependency

Dependency hearings are the most powerful court proceedings connected with a child. Once CPS intervenes and the juvenile court takes jurisdiction, grandparents and grandchildren are locked into the system for a defined period of time. Decisions are taken out of the hands of the family and placed in the hands of the court. Parents and grandparents lose control of the situation. In most states the dependency system has exclusive jurisdiction over issues of child custody; it overrules all other courts, including family law and probate. This means that while the case is active in the dependency process, no other court can make decisions about the child. In other words, once your grandchild goes into the system, you are married to the courts for as long as the process lasts. For a grandparent, this can pose serious problems:

• *The dependency process is a mystery.* Cases are usually closed except to the parties involved—generally, the child, the parents, the child welfare agency, and in some cases, interested relatives and other supportive persons. This means that the public and the press cannot typically come into these courtrooms the way they may come into criminal and civil courts. Unless you've already been involved in a dependency court case, you're not likely to know what to expect. A lot goes on in a dependency courtroom, and it all seems to happen quickly. What you see is just a fragment of what happens; the 15 minutes you spend in front of a judge represents hours of attorney time. And court personnel often talk in legal shorthand that can change from district to district.

• *Dependency can be a nightmare of bureaucracy.* Systems are systems. They are big and unwieldy. And it can seem like everyone in this system is working against one another. Because caseloads are high, communication in the system is challenging, and sometimes critical information doesn't reach the presiding judge. One child welfare agency director describes dependency as "a mass custody suit where six to eight different interests are represented."

• *Dependency is relentless.* Although there are state and federal timelines for when certain hearings must take place, courts occasionally waive these deadlines—for a range of reasons—and the process can drag on, sometimes for years.

Grandparents repeatedly get lost and overwhelmed in the maze of steps and hearings that make up the dependency process. Here, as everywhere, knowledge is your best tool. It is important to know how things work and what is possible. It is also important to remember that all these professionals—social workers, attorneys, judges—do share a common goal. That goal is "to support, nurture, reunify, and heal families," says attorney Leslie Heimov, executive director of the Children's Law Center of California. "We want children to go home and be with parents...safely.

And when they can't go home, we want them to be with extended family."[3]

DEPENDENCY: STEP BY STEP

Dependency law is extensive and complex. This discussion is only a general blueprint of the process; it is designed as a tool to help you ask questions about the laws and regulations in your own state. Although every stage of the dependency process has various possible outcomes, each explanation given below assumes, for simplicity's sake, that the child has been removed from the home and placed with relatives. The schedule used in this discussion reflects Los Angeles County procedures. Your own state laws may outline more steps, different names, and a different timeline. And please remember that this chapter is meant to offer insight, but it cannot replace sound legal advice. Talk with an attorney about your specific situation.

The Call

A parent is arrested or injured, and no one is around to take the children. A child is left alone in an apartment for hours. A teacher suspects a student is being abused at home. The dependency process starts with a call to CPS about a child who is suspected of being abandoned, neglected, or abused. CPS then sends out an emergency response social worker to investigate the situation.

Anyone can call CPS about a child at risk, including clergy, neighbors, and family members. Some states also have a list of "mandated reporters." Mandated reporters are individuals who are required by law to report any suspicion of child abuse or neglect (for example, teachers, doctors, therapists, and child care providers). How soon the investigation takes place depends on the nature of the allegation. A call about suspected abuse generally receives more immediate attention than a call about neglect. Even if the caller can provide an address but no name, CPS must respond.

Depending on what the social worker finds, one of several things can happen:

- The referral can be dismissed for lack of evidence.
- The parents may agree to seek counseling, rehabilitation, or other services to correct the problem, and the child remains in the home, in which case the dependency court may or may not get involved.
- The child may be considered to be "at risk" and removed from parental custody, in which case the dependency court will get involved.

Of course, what social workers actually find during an investigation often depends on when they visit and how thorough they are. A worker who makes an immediate unannounced visit, for instance, will often see a different picture than one who makes an appointment. Even a day's notice can give neglectful parents time to clean the house, stock the refrigerator, and generally make a better impression.

The Pickup

If a social worker (or police officer) finds enough evidence to indicate that a child is at risk of abuse or neglect in the home, the child will be taken into protective custody. Some states may release a child into the care of a relative if one shows up with proof of relationship and a clean background check. At this point the referral can either be dismissed or referred to the dependency court through a "petition of dependency" (see below). However, if no one comes to take the child or if for some reason CPS won't release him, the social worker must refer the case to the dependency court for a hearing. During this time the child could be inaccessible to the family.

■ WHAT YOU NEED TO KNOW

Keep track of your grandchildren. If you know they have been picked up by CPS, be persistent in locating them. Although federal law requires CPS to look for, notify, and consider all available adult relatives before placing a child in foster care, this may not always happen in a timely fashion. Be sure to take birth certificates or something that proves your relationship to the children, especially if their last name is different from yours. Your actions may not prevent the dependency process from kicking into gear, but if CPS will release the children to you, it will make it easier for you to get placement down the line. At the very least, let the social worker know you are interested in placement or future visitation.

The Petition

A petition of dependency is the legal document that tells a judge why the social worker thinks the court should intervene to protect the child. In essence, it is the state's formal allegation against the parents for the abuse and neglect of a minor, and it formally requests that the child be made a dependent of the court. The petition must be filed within *48 court hours* (that is, two working days) of the child being taken into protective custody.[4] It includes whatever facts the child welfare agency believes will support its claims and identifies the sections of the law under which the parents are accused; these accusations are important because they determine which programs the parents will have to complete in order to regain custody of the child. For instance, if the petition claims the child has been physically abused but there are no allegations of drug use, the court may send a parent to parenting class or individual counseling, but it will not send the parents to drug treatment.

The Detention Hearing

The detention hearing (sometimes known as "arraignment and detention," "initial hearing," "shelter care hearing," or "temporary custody hearing") is the first judicial proceeding in a dependency case, the hearing that sets the case in motion. This hearing generally takes place within three court days of the child being removed from parental custody. It is a quick hearing, sometimes without a thorough investigation beforehand and with just a brief report from the emergency response worker.

At the detention hearing the parents are formally informed of the reason the child was taken into temporary custody and of the allegations against them. At that hearing, CPS provides a detention packet to the court and attorneys that lists the allegations of abuse or neglect against the parents and a report that outlines details about the family situation that led to the children's removal from the home.

This is also the stage where parents are informed of their right to an attorney. If they cannot afford one, some states will appoint one free of charge. Some states also appoint an attorney for the child—someone who specializes in representing children in dependency court. Other states use the same attorney who represents CPS (sometimes called the Department of Social Services, or DSS) to represent the child.

The parents, the children, CPS, and their attorneys have a right to be present at the hearing. Caregivers, relatives, and friends often attend. Whether they are allowed into the courtroom may depend on the specific rules of that particular jurisdiction or courtroom.

Two issues are decided at the detention hearing stage: (1) how the parents will respond to the allegations and (2) whether there is enough evidence to detain the child in temporary custody until the court determines whether the allegations in the petition are true. If the parents do not dispute the charges, the case will go on to a disposition hearing. However, if the parents deny the charges, the case will move on to mediation or trial.

In determining whether it is necessary to take a child into temporary custody, the court will consider the report provided by CPS as well as legal arguments from the attorneys regarding the need for a child to remain out of the home or whether safeguards could be put in place so that the child could be returned. In the event a child is not returned home, attorneys often make requests to let children live with relatives or close family friends. If a child has not been placed with a relative or close family friend prior to the detention hearing, the judge will often order an investigation of a possible caregiver, the members of the caregiver's household, and the caregiver's home. A further court date is then set to address placement of the children in that home.

■ WHAT YOU NEED TO KNOW

The detention hearing is a critical hearing. If you are aware of it, try to show up. You might not be able to go inside the courtroom for the hearing—these hearings are confidential—but you can let the court officers, social workers, or child's attorney know, for the record and before the hearing, that you are a grandparent and want to be a resource. Federal law gives preference to placing children with relatives, but the court has to know you exist. Also, preferential consideration does not guarantee placement. CPS must run a background and criminal check on you and assess your home before they can let you take your grandchild home.

If the court won't consider you for placement, you might be able to request visitation while your grandchild is in the care of another relative or in foster care.

Mediation and/or Trial

The decision-making phase of the dependency process involves mediation and/or trial. This is the stage where the court decides whether or not the allegations against the parents are true and, if so, whether the state will assume legal custody of the child. These determinations are generally made in a "jurisdictional hearing" (or trial), but some states try to avoid the need for a trial by settling the case through mediation.

Mediation Stage

Some states insert a mediation stage (sometimes called a "pretrial hearing" or a "pretrial resolution conference") between the detention and jurisdictional hearings. At this hearing, CPS submits a report that contains a more thorough investigation of the allegations. The report includes interviews of family members, victims, and other witnesses that may be used at trial. It also contains the recommended case plan outlining the services needed to help families address the abuse issues that brought the case to court. This is the state's attempt to settle a case without going to trial. Sometimes the allegations in the petition can be proven untrue and the case is dismissed. Sometimes a parent is willing to admit to the charges in the petition, or the petition can be amended to reflect charges a parent *will* admit to. For instance, a father may have earlier denied the allegations of drug abuse but by the mediation stage he may admit to occasional cocaine use. If a settlement is reached, the case could go directly to a "disposition hearing" (see below), sometimes even the same day. However, if the parents continue to deny all allegations, the case goes to a jurisdictional hearing, or trial.

Trial Stage

If a settlement is not reached through mediation or if a state does not provide mediation services, the case goes into the trial phase of the dependency process. This trial is also known as the adjudication, or jurisdictional hearing, where witnesses testify and evidence is admitted for the court to review. CPS is responsible for presenting evidence that the child has been abused or neglected. The child's attorney, having conducted an independent investigation of the allegations, then presents evidence supporting his or her assessment of the case. The attorney for the parents questions the evidence and presents counterevidence. Finally, the judge decides if any charges in the petition against the parents are true and whether to make the child a dependent of the court. If the court finds the entire petition is not true, or the allegations are true but do not rise to the level of abuse or neglect, the case is dismissed and the child is returned to the home. If the court finds that any portion of the petition is true, the case is set for a disposition hearing.

■ WHAT YOU NEED TO KNOW

It is important to understand which charges are proven or admitted at the trial stage because they will be important at the disposition hearing, when the court decides what plan the parents must follow to regain custody of the child. For instance, if a petition claims a parent has a drug problem and is physically abusive but the judge doesn't see enough evidence to prove drug abuse, the case plan generally will not include drug rehabilitation services. However, if additional proof appears later on, CPS can often make new allegations or amend the petition, so make your grandchild's social worker aware of what you know—and can prove—as the case goes along.

The Disposition Hearing

If any of the allegations against the parents are judged true, the case goes to a disposition hearing. This is where the court decides what to do to both protect the child and help the parents regain custody. At or before the disposition hearing the child's social worker submits a report on the status of the case and a case plan with recommendations about where the child should live, whether the child can live with the parents, and if not, how often the parents should visit or call, and what services should be offered to the children and the parents to improve conditions in the home and facilitate the return of the child to the parents.

The judge considers the social worker's report and recommendations, as well as evidence and arguments from other parties, before making a decision on the case. Final court orders typically include a "reunification case plan," which documents what conditions the parents must fulfill in order to regain custody of the child, a visitation schedule, and a decision on placement for the child. The placement plan may include sending the child home with a parent under CPS supervision or placing the child in the home of a relative or a close family friend, or in a foster home. It is always the goal to place siblings together whenever possible; however, if there are circumstances preventing siblings from being placed together, a visitation plan is outlined to establish or maintain the sibling bonds.[5]

Periodic Reviews

Once the child has been placed with a relative or foster parents and reunification services have been offered to the parents, there will be periodic hearings (also known as "administrative case reviews," "judicial reviews," "family reunification review hearings," and "dependency status reviews") to review the family's progress. These reviews are conducted every six months by either the court or the child welfare agency and consider both the case and the case plan. Questions such as the following are addressed: Is the case plan being followed? Are the parents regularly visiting the children? Are visits going well? How are the parents progressing? Are they testing as required? What are the results of those tests? Have the parents been attending all court-ordered classes? Do they understand the issues in the case? Does the child need additional services? When might the child return to parental custody? If by the second review it seems unlikely that the child will return home, a permanent plan may be established. If the parents are doing well but are not quite ready to resume custody, the court can grant a six-month extension before deciding on the permanent plan.

■ WHAT YOU NEED TO KNOW

Although relative caregivers may be entitled to receive notification of each review hearing in advance, they are rarely notified in time, if at all. Since you know these reviews take place every six months, try to keep track of when they are scheduled. Let the judge, the child's lawyer, and the social worker know that you want to be informed of these hearings, and try to attend. Be prepared to talk about how you are facilitating the reunification plan if you are asked and to provide comments and observations about the child's reactions to parental visits. This is another place where careful documentation can be helpful. If you are monitoring parents' visits, note the times, dates, places, and quality of the family visits. Also, keep records of all legal documents, bills, correspondence, and contacts with the lawyer, the social worker, the court, and the parents. If you submit information for the court, make copies for all the attorneys involved to make sure everyone reads it. (Note: In California, caregivers may file a Caregiver Information Form with the court. This form enables you to provide medical, dental, psychological, and educational information about the child, as well as anything else you would like to relay regarding parental visits, progress on reunification, etc. Ask if anything like this is available in your state.)

Permanency Planning Hearing

Federal law requires that a permanent plan for each child who enters the dependency system be established within 6 to 18 months[*] from the date of the original placement (unless the parent has been institutionalized or incarcerated during the family reunification time period. If so, in some jurisdictions the court can extend services to a maximum of twenty-four months).[6] At this point the child must either be safely returned to the parents or family reunification services will be terminated.

If the court does not return the child to parental custody, it then sets a separate hearing to determine which permanent plan is best for the child:

---

[*]Family reunification can be extended to 18 months if, at the 12-month hearing, the court finds substantial probability that the child will be returned to the parents within the next 6 months.

adoption, guardianship, or another planned permanency living arrangement (formerly called "long-term foster care").

Adoption often has the highest priority because it is the most permanent solution. If the court identifies adoption as the permanent plan, the court will then terminate parental rights and free the child for adoption.

In California, the court can decide not to terminate parental rights under several circumstances:

- The child is living with a relative who doesn't want to adopt but is committed to the child and is willing to become a legal guardian.
- The court finds that terminating parental rights is not in the child's best interest because

    1. Parents have maintained visitation and a parental relationship and role such that it would be detrimental to sever that relationship.
    2. The child is 12 years or older and objects to adoption.
    3. There would be a substantial interference with a sibling relationship that would be detrimental to the child to the point of outweighing the benefit of adoption.

In such cases, guardianship would be the preferred plan. Guardianship only lasts until the child is 18 years old, and it can be terminated before then. Long-term foster care is the least stable option. This "permanency planning" hearing must occur within 120 days of termination of family reunification services.[7]

◼ WHAT YOU NEED TO KNOW

You don't have to adopt your grandchild. While the courts do look at adoption as a first choice, there are reasons grandparents may not want to adopt a grandchild: They may not be ready to give up on their adult children, or they may feel that their age, health, or finances might rule out adoption. Guardianship is a valid alternative, and many states have federally subsidized funding programs for relatives—Kinship Guardian Assistance Programs, sometimes called KinGAP—to help facilitate kinship guardianship as a permanent plan for children in relative foster care.

"The truth is that the court looks at the relative caregiver very differently than they look at a nonrelated caregiver," says attorney Pamela Mohr. "They realize there is a familial obligation. Even if the kid is not legally your kid, the kid is your grandkid and will be your grandkid for the rest of your life. They aren't worried about your just abandoning the child."[8] (See "Adoption" in Chapter 10 and "Adoption Assistance Program" in Chapter 12.)

However, if you choose to adopt at a later date, as legal guardian, you may ask the court to reopen the case and set a hearing to terminate parental rights in order to free the child for adoption.

■ HOW TO COPE

• *Start early!* It is critical that you express your concern for your grandchild as early in the dependency process as possible, especially if you want the child placed with you. Although federal law requires CPS to identify family resources and notify relatives, this may not always be fully accomplished or done in a timely fashion. There may not be enough time to look for family. Parents may be uncooperative about supplying names and phone numbers. Some social workers may simply neglect to look for or interview relatives. Unfortunately, if too much time passes, the court may rule out relative placement altogether. For example, the child may have bonded with foster parents, who may be considering adoption, and the court may be unwilling to disrupt the situation. If you cannot locate your grandchild but suspect that she is in the system, contact child welfare in the child's last known location and let them know that you are a resource.

Of course, a preference for placing children with relatives doesn't guarantee that placement. The court must first evaluate your ability to provide a safe, secure, and stable home for the child. Among other things, it will also consider your willingness to support visitation and reunification with the parent, whether or not you have a criminal record, and whether previous allegations of child abuse have been made against you.

Even if you can't get placement early on, you can ask for visitation. This at least would allow you to continue your involvement in your grandchild's life, a fact that could be important if you later seek placement or custody. In fact, don't hesitate to let the social worker and the court know if you are willing to take your grandchild on a permanent basis in the event that the parents cannot fulfill the reunification requirements. The sooner you express your interest, the more likelihood you have of being considered.

• *Attend hearings!* Once your grandchild is in the system, attend every hearing that you can. You may not be permitted into the courtroom, but let the bailiff, the child's attorney, or the court clerk know that you are there, that you are a grandparent, and that you are interested in place-ment or visitation. The fact that there exists a real person who is willing to take a child can sometimes affect the judge's decision. You can also write a letter to the judge. If you do, send copies to all the attorneys involved and keep it simple.

• *Ask about standing.* "Standing" is the right to participate in a case as a party, which means you are entitled to receive notice of hearings and to present evidence and may be entitled to be represented by an attor-ney. Although rules of the court often change from county to county in terms of who may speak in court, when they may do so, and under what circumstances, the parties who have standing in a dependency case are generally the parents, the child, and the child welfare agency. Grandpar-ents and other relatives typically do not have standing in a dependency case; they may not even be permitted in the courtroom. However, some states will allow a person who has raised and provided for a child for some time to qualify as a de facto parent, that is, a parent "in actuality" or a substitute parent. This de facto parent, whether related to the child or not, may be entitled to standing and, in some cases, may be assigned a court-appointed attorney. However, you could have to hire a private attor-ney in order to prove de facto parent status.

Some states allow relatives limited participation in a dependency case without full standing.[9] Judges also have the authority to let you in the courtroom if they want to hear what you have to say. Keep asking ques-tions until you know exactly what kind of involvement you are entitled to in your court system.

• *Behave yourself in court.* Grandparents have an image problem in court. In their zeal to protect their grandchildren (and their frustra-tion with the system), they often argue with court clerks, attorneys, and even judges, attempting to clarify the danger of the situation and the need to move quickly. Despite their best intentions this approach often backfires. Grandparents may become known as troublemakers and find that court personnel are less likely to listen to them. In some instances, cases may even be delayed. You will have more success if you follow two rules:

1. Be gracious with court officials, from clerks and bailiffs to the judge in your case. Remember that when you deal with the court system you are asking for help; you don't score points by making demands. Remember, too, that this is their "house," as it were, and you must follow their rules.

2. Be polite in court. Don't interrupt or blurt out comments. Try to stay calm; avoid arguing with the parents in front of the judge. Cooperate with your attorney, if you have one. Above all, don't argue with the judge. (For more on court behavior see, "A Word about Judges," below.)

• *Be prepared for delays.* From the moment the child is removed, a clock starts ticking. According to federal law, a permanent plan must be established for a child no later than 18 months from the date of the original placement. However, it may not always happen that way. Marjorie Brown's granddaughter was six months old when she was placed with Marjorie and was almost three by the time a permanent plan was established. Various factors contribute to these delays. Rising caseloads make scheduling difficult at every stage. Hearings may be continued over several dates to allow for further investigation or psychological evaluations. Illness on the part of attorneys, judges, or key participants can delay proceedings. And in certain situations—for example, the parents are doing well but need more time to complete the case plan—reunification services might be extended an additional six months.

• *Support family reunification.* Parents may be entitled to as little or as much as six to 24 months of reunification services (depending on the state and the circumstances).[10] If you wish to have your grandchild placed with you, you must keep your feelings about the parents private and work actively toward reuniting the parents with the child—even if you think reunification is the most horrible thing that could happen to your grandchild. If you cannot support reunification, the court may not place the child with you. It may not be able to. And if you speak or act against the parents while the child is living with you, social services can remove him.

Of course, that doesn't mean you must let a parent see a child when he or she shows up intoxicated on your doorstep, but it does mean you must do everything else to actively encourage reunification: Advocate not just for the child but for the *family*. Understand the case plan and make sure that services are truly offered from the beginning. Encourage the parent to attend all required classes. Ask for the rules and schedule for visitation and cooperate fully. Document in writing your efforts to support reunification: how often parents visit, how visits go, and how your grand-child is doing.

"If parents are too helpless, hopeless, or not sophisticated enough to navigate the system, and they don't receive services," says Heimov, "you could find yourself in an unnecessary battle 12–18 months down the road. And in that scenario, nobody wins."[11] However, if services are offered from the start, and if everyone—Mom, Dad, the kids, and even you, if appropriate—gets the services they need, then by the end of reunification, the next step can be clear: either the children can go home safely—and you can return to being supportive grandparents—or the parents are truly not ready, and it's really time for a permanent plan.

HOTLINES ARE NOT ALWAYS HELP LINES

Claire Powers called a child abuse hotline to help her granddaughter; in the end she lost her. The system went out, found Mom, and pulled her back into the picture. And Mom came running. To quote one family law judge, "The most disinterested parent in the world becomes the most interested when someone tries to interfere with their God-given, constitutionally protected right to parent."

But this is not the only reason to avoid hotlines. If you call a child abuse hotline on your adult child and he or she finds out, you can find yourself trapped in the system. If your grandchild is removed from a parent, he or she may do everything possible to keep the child out of your home. Some parents will even lie; they may say that you were an abusive parent, an alcoholic—anything to make you pay for making the call. "It's like calling the cops on your daughter or son," explains attorney Ted Youmans. "You're probably not going to be befriending the kid. You'll be alienating yourself right from the start, and the system will probably treat you with alienation as the one who complained."[12]

Remember, anything that interferes with reunification is suspect, and a bad relationship between parent and grandparent is a red flag to social workers and to the court. Judges are wary of grandparents whose children say, "I hate them. I can't get along with them. I can't visit my kids at their house; they interfere." Those grandparents might not get placement.

HOW TO AVOID INVOLVEMENT WITH THE SYSTEM

Most grandparents involved with the dependency system had no choice in the matter—a social worker showed up on their doorstep with their grandchildren in tow or the hospital held a drug-exposed infant in protective custody. In other words, the system arrived with the child. Some grandparents, however, have many chances to bypass government involvement if they realize there is a problem and know enough to think ahead.

• *Keep track of your grandchildren.* Do so especially when parents have problems. Offer to watch your grandchildren occasionally. Visit and call often, if the parents will let you. If there has been a problem in the past, let schools and local hospitals know that you are available as an emergency contact. Once children are in the foster care system, it can be difficult and heartbreaking to try to get them out.

• *Keep track of your adult children.* Do so even with those who don't have children yet. I have talked to grandparents from various states who tell me that they didn't even know they had a grandchild until the child was four or five years old and already in foster care. If a parent is arrested without someone available to take the child, children's services will probably take over. Keep the lines of communication open and active, especially when you're in another state. If your adult child has any responsible friends, give them your telephone number in case of emergency. Because my parents lived nearby, they were immediately able to take in my nephew when my sister died. However, had Nikki died in another city, Kevin might have gone into a foster home before anyone in the family knew it. Furthermore, since Nikki didn't have a will, child welfare might not even have known that Kevin had grandparents who could take him. The bottom line is that keeping track of the parent is the only way to keep track of the child.

• *Think ahead.* In case of emergency, how could you prove your relationship to your grandchild? Do you have your adult child's birth certificate? Do you have your grandchild's birth certificate? If your own child is the father, did he sign the birth certificate? If you are on good terms with the parents, in case of illness or accident, could you get a signed statement proving your relationship? Unless a grandchild is old enough to identify you, proving your relationship can be complicated, particularly if the child has a different last name from yours. Planning ahead can save time, heartache, and money in the event of an emergency.

• *Consider guardianship.* If the grandchildren are with you and their parents have vanished, consider becoming their guardian. The dependency system will make you jump through legal hoops. Social workers will conduct visits once a month, adding to the stress and tension you are already experiencing. However, if you go into probate, you're in control, not the system. (For more on guardianship, see Chapter 10.)

WHEN YOU MIGHT WANT THE SYSTEM INVOLVED

There are actually reasons you might want the system involved in your grandchild's case: the child's safety and your own peace of mind. Perhaps you cannot afford to apply for legal guardianship. Perhaps your family situation or personal history would prevent a judge from giving you custody. Perhaps your grandchild isn't with you, and the situation is too dangerous to wait for a guardianship hearing. This is a time when you may actually want to call CPS. Sometimes *anything*—even foster care—is better than leaving a grandchild in an abusive home. It's not a perfect solution, but it can be the lesser evil.

Understand, however, that if you are the one to call the police or CPS, there is a possibility the child will not be placed with you. A lot depends on your background check, what your son or daughter says about you, and whether or not you live in the same state. Still, sometimes it is worth involving the system to protect a child who is at risk.

WHEN THE SYSTEM WON'T GET INVOLVED

It may seem to you that social workers and judges are just hovering in the doorways ready to snatch up any child who may be in danger, that after one call the child will be whisked away to safety. At least that is the belief of hopeful grandparents who call child abuse hotlines. Actually, it's not always true. Sometimes the system won't get involved in a case and that can be an equal source of frustration to some grandparents.

There are times when calling CPS won't do anything. Allegations of child abuse and neglect require witnesses and evidence, sometimes physical proof. This can infuriate grandparents who know of the kind of abuse that doesn't leave marks. Emotional abuse may not show on a child's body, but the scars are often more difficult to heal. Moreover, the legal definitions of abuse and neglect not only vary from state to state but are interpreted differently from social worker to social worker and from one judge to the next. Furthermore, leaving children with grandparents, family, or friends is rarely considered desertion or abandonment. Child welfare agencies regularly turn away children who are living with relatives without parental interference; their reasoning is that the child is not in danger.

Generally, a grandparent in this situation has three choices: continue to care for the child informally, return the child to the parents and wait until she is abused or neglected, or file for private guardianship. As we saw in Chapter 10, guardianship offers greater protection.

A WORD ABOUT SOCIAL WORKERS

In the field of social work, as in most professions, there are good workers and bad ones. Which kind you get is the luck of the draw, but the difference is often immediately clear. Good social workers are thorough. When they investigate a case, they really investigate. They talk to the children; they look for bruises and ask for explanations; they study a home for things that signal neglect. Good social workers are supportive. They listen to your concerns, return phone calls, and link you up with resources and information. They let you know what kind of financial assistance is available to your grandchild and how you can apply for it. Some will even refer you to a support group. In fact, many of our families are referred to us through their social workers.

Bad social workers are a nightmare. They range from the poorly informed to the actively heartless, from the ones who give you incorrect information about department regulations and government benefits to the ones who have a fixed prejudice against grandparents. One social worker, who didn't know me, talked to me about a grandmother I know. "She's ruining everyone's life," she told me. "I can't deal with her." She also called her "crazy" and "invasive." This attitude is a common problem for grandparents. Many social workers see them as picking fights with their children out of vengeance—"hollerin' wolf" as one grandmother calls it.[13] In fact, the war stories are legendary. I received a letter from a woman whose daughter died, leaving her with three small children to care for. Like many grandparents, she discovered that it is difficult to feed and clothe growing children on a fixed income. Her social worker told her she was expected to "cut coupons and shop at Goodwill, just like every-one else on welfare." When one young woman placed her two children with her mother, social services removed them because the grandmother was "too old." Beth and Alan Grafton had a fight on their hands to get cus-tody of their grandchildren after their son-in-law murdered their daughter. The reason? Beth would cry when she discussed her daughter's death. The worker assigned to the case decided that Grandma "wasn't grieving properly" and recommended against custody.

If you are raising your grandchildren, you will, most likely, have to work with social workers. You find them at each stage of the game, from intake workers to long-term case workers. Moreover, sometimes everything can depend on the decision of a social worker. As one young woman admitted to Claire Powers, "I look at 30 minutes in this child's life and play God." So, some words of advice . . .

• *Be nice to social workers.* After all, you want them on your side. Social workers have great power: They present information to judges; sometimes they're also your only source of information. Work with them. Endear yourself to them, if you can. Don't make demands. And remember that you share the same goal: the safety and well-being of the child.

• *Use understanding.* It is easier to work with people if you under-stand what obstacles they are fighting. Social workers are as much at the mercy of a bureaucratic system as are children and grandparents. Social workers in some large cities oversee unusually high caseloads. They are often undertrained and underpaid—and they burn out quickly. An official in one city reported that half his staff had been working less than a year.[14] Between being new on the job and having case overload, many social workers don't have time to keep up with changes in the law, track available resources, or even listen in the ways they want to. "It's hard, as a social worker, to service the families the way that we would like to because we have so many clients," admits one social worker. "We're not really capable of doing a lot of one-on-one work with our families." Says grandparent activist Ethel Dunn, "You go into social services [and] they are in chaos, not because everyone in the social service system is a poor social worker but it's simply that they don't have the wherewithal to do the job they're given."[15]

- *Communicate regularly with your grandchild's social worker.* Open communication and a good rapport with your grandchild's social worker are key to making sure he gets everything he needs. Try to establish clear expectations about what information needs to be shared and what rules and procedures must be followed. Remember, you are both advocating for the safety, well-being, and development of your grandchild. Communication can be damaged if a social worker thinks you're violating rules or placing a child at risk. If, despite your best efforts, a social worker is unresponsive or hard to work with, you can contact his supervisor.

- *Tell specific facts.* Tell your grandchild's social worker what you saw with your own eyes, not what you heard from other people. If you can, offer witnesses; they may be viewed as less biased.

- *Try not to make it personal.* There are few things that are more personal than the fate of those we love. But if you are involved in the dependency system, you must try to understand and play by its rules. For instance, try to remember that assessing your home is a legal requirement designed to protect the children, not to disrespect your family. If your grandkids had to live with strangers, what questions would you want the social worker to ask them? They need to ask the same questions of you. It is understandably scary—there is always that fear of not being approved—but the more you can understand the reasons for licensing standards, court dates, visiting agreements, etc., the less personal it will feel.

• *Keep the mandates in mind.* The truth is that you and your grand-child's social worker share a commitment to making sure your grand-child is safe, well, and in a stable living arrangement. The difference is that, for you, these goals are driven by love; for the social worker, they are defined by law. Child protection and the dependency system have clearly, and legally, defined goals: child safety, child well-being, and per-manency. What that means is that your grandchild will not be reabused or neglected, that his needs will be met, and he will grow up in a safe, nur-turing, *and permanent* home and family. Reunification with the parents is the first goal for permanency, provided the child is safe. A permanent living arrangement with a relative is the preferred choice after that. The more you can understand and stay focused on these outcomes, even in this language, the easier it will be for you and the social worker to col-laborate on your grandchild's behalf.

• *Remember whose case it is.* You may, as a grandparent, talk about "my case" and "my social worker," and it can certainly feel that way. You are trying to protect your grandchild from her parents and from a system that seems to have anything but your grandchild's best interests at heart. Grandparents have a lot riding on their social worker and their case. A good social worker may understand this, but he won't see it the same way. He can't. He is your grandchild's social worker, handling your grandchild's case. His job is to protect the child's interests and, if possible, return her to the custody of her parents.

Remember, not every social worker who disagrees with a grandpar-ent is a bad social worker. Not every child who cannot be with his par-ents should be with his grandparents. There are grandparents who really should not have their grandchildren because of medical or psychological problems. Some children may be better off in a foster home if there is no other relative to take them.

A WORD ABOUT JUDGES

The judge is the wild card in any legal situation. Judges don't write laws, but they interpret them. Judges don't investigate cases, but they rule on them. In a limited time frame and with selective information a judge makes binding decisions about a child's future, and each decision is as individual as the judge who made it. All judges are rule-bound, but some follow the rules more closely than others. As attorneys, they are taught to think unemotionally, to think about "best interest" in legal terms. However, there are those who appreciate the emotional realities of these cases and will listen to the experts who understand them, such as psychologists and child care professionals.

Some judges can seem terribly unfair and inconsistent—like the one who let nine-year-old Travis Jackson testify against his father for killing his mother but wouldn't let him choose to live with his grandparents. Others are plainly insensitive. "Some grandparents have a need to steal their grandchildren," one judge told a grandmother. "Is that the case here?" I have even heard about a probate judge who turned to an attorney and barked, "What's all this about 'bonding?' We're not talking about real estate here!"

On the other hand, I also hear stories of judges who are not only sensitive to grandparents' and grandchildren's interests but understand what is at stake. An unorthodox judge in Arizona settled a dispute in which everyone in a large family was fighting bitterly over two grandchildren. The judge had every person involved in the case come into the courtroom and forbade anyone to speak. Then she had the children brought in. She watched to see whom they ran to—it turned out to be the grandparents—and awarded them custody.[16] "Grandparents are the safety net for the children of today," acknowledged one presiding judge in California.[17]

For the most part, however, few judges really think about grandparent concerns. Part of the reason is that they often cannot. Judges interpret the laws but they are limited by them. According to the law, once a child's safety is ensured, the next goal is the reunification of child and parent. "I can't take a child from a parent because I'd like to," said another California judge. "I can't even take a child from a parent because down deep in my heart I really want to. I can only interfere in a parent–child relationship if to continue that relationship would be a detriment to the child and to place the child with a nonparent is in the child's best interest. It's not a balancing act; it's a dual-focus question."[18]

Another problem, however, is that judges, like social workers, have impossible caseloads. They may not have time to read all the critical documents involved in a case, and they may come to court unprepared. Their decisions can reflect that. Also, they are often dependent on the information they get from social workers and attorneys.

If you find yourself in the dependency system or if you apply for guardianship or adoption or even if you appeal an administrative decision about government aid, you may find yourself facing a judge. If you do and you are given the opportunity to speak in court, there are a few principles you may want to keep in mind:

- *Be respectful.* Dress appropriately for court, and be on your best behavior.
- *Be informed.* There are some situations in which grandparents may represent themselves in court, such as in visitation or guardianship hearings in certain states. If you are in such a situation, you are expected to be as familiar with the laws and procedures that affect your case as an attorney is. If you represent yourself, educate yourself.
- *Be clear.* If you do speak in court, make your statements short and to the point. Stick to facts. Ask the judge if he or she has any questions.
- *Go through proper channels.* It is the judge who decides if anyone other than a party to the case may be heard, and some don't want to hear from relatives in the courtroom. If you need to communicate something to the judge, let the child's attorney know or ask the child's social worker to attach a letter to the court report. Some courts also use Caregiver Information Forms. Be forewarned, however, that anything the court looks at is given to all parties and is not private.
- *Be a part of the solution.* Judges welcome information and constructive ideas that serve the child's best interests. Whenever possible, try to resolve your differences out of court, then ask the judge to make an order based on your agreement.

And remember, no two courtrooms are the same. Everything that happens in a particular courtroom is filtered through the perspective of that particular judge. Which judge you get is often the luck of the draw. However, it can set the tone for your grandchild's entire case.

12

Government Aid
and Public Assistance

A single adult eats differently than a family. The food bill at least tripled. The water bill shot up. Instead of one shower a day, I now had five. Toilet paper? I thought they were eating it when they came. About the only thing that did go down was my gas because I could never go anywhere.

—*Grandmother raising four grandkids*

Raising a grandchild is not only an emotional and legal challenge but a financial one as well. Some grandparents deplete their savings, take out second mortgages on their homes, and even do without their own necessities in order to provide for their grandchildren. Few think about government aid. Many grandparents simply don't know that financial assistance is available to them; often this is because they have their grandchildren on an informal basis. However, even when children are placed by child protective services (CPS) or the court, many social workers neglect to tell grandparents and relatives that they are entitled to aid for a child.

Remember Leah Croft? She was already raising her daughter's six-year-old twins when another grandchild, Josh, arrived at her house—late at night, unexpected, and in the arms of a social worker. Leah was a single, working grandmother on a moderate salary. The twins had lived with her for four years, and she had stretched her limited budget to accommodate them. She didn't know the twins were entitled to welfare benefits, so she had never asked for them. Then the new baby arrived, and the expenses nearly took her over the edge financially. Although Josh was placed with her by CPS, no one from the agency told her that he might be eligible for foster care benefits. Furthermore, after Leah found out about and applied for foster care benefits, no one told her she could get welfare assistance for the baby while she waited. For five months she put diapers and baby supplies on her credit card, because that was all she had. Leah eventually received retroactive benefits for the months she waited, but she is still paying the interest those credit card charges incurred.

Lack of information is the toughest financial problem you may face as a grandparent; it keeps you out of the game entirely. If you don't know, you can't ask, and if you can't ask, you may not get the help you need and deserve. The good news is that government assistance is available to you, primarily through programs that support dependent children. Just because you are caring for your grandchildren does not mean you have an obligation to support them—even if you are their legal guardian. Only parents (biological or adoptive) have that responsibility. The government recognizes this, which is why programs like foster care were developed. Although grandparents fall into a gray area between parents and foster parents, there are a number of assistance programs that may apply to you and your grandchildren, from welfare and foster care benefits to social security and adoption assistance.

THE DIFFICULTIES OF WORKING WITH THE GOVERNMENT

Government aid means working with the government. You may find yourself navigating a maze of bureaucracy, poor information, and seemingly unfair rules. You may also struggle with the social stigma of welfare or the inequalities of the foster care system. The very agencies designed to support your grandchildren can seem like more of a hindrance than a help. But advance knowledge can often prevent problems, and it will always prepare you to face them.

Misinformation

After lack of information, the most common problem grandparents face in dealing with government agencies is poor information. You may ask the right questions, but the answers you get are either half true or completely wrong. The reason is that social and welfare workers don't always know the right answers. They may be undertrained or unaware of changes in the law. Perhaps they don't understand how a particular program applies to grandparent families. For instance, you yourself may not be eligible for welfare, but your grandchild may be. But if no one tells you, you won't know.

Government employees are rarely malicious but may be ill informed. Unfortunately, some of them will swear their poor information is the gospel truth. Be cautious when you deal with social workers and eligibility workers. Ask questions to clarify what they tell you. Learn what you can about local rules and regulations, and contact other grandparents and support groups to compare notes. Accurate information is your key to government assistance.

Bureaucracy

Dealing with government agencies is rarely a cut-and-dried experience. It can mean long lines, extensive paperwork, and bureaucratic mistakes. You may wait in three different lines at the welfare office just to get a packet of forms, then wait in another line to schedule an appointment. If you work, you may have to take the day off in order to attend an interview. If your grandchildren have to be there, you'll need to cart toys and lunch along for them. It could turn into a whole-day affair. This is particularly difficult for grandparents who are disabled and cannot sit for long periods of time. Calling isn't better. Because many eligibility workers have restricted telephone hours, it can take days to connect with them.

If you are having a difficult time reaching an eligibility worker, you may want to talk to her supervisor. First, document the times you try to call and the names of people you speak with. Write letters when you can (and keep copies for yourself). Then, if you do have to go over the worker's head, you have proof of what occurred.

Long lines and mistakes are an inevitable part of dealing with the government. All you can do is be alert for errors and be patient with the rest—and try to do something nice for yourself when you get home!

Unequal Benefits

There are two key assistance programs that grandparents and relatives get involved with: welfare assistance and foster care. Both provide cash assistance to needy children, but foster care offers substantially higher benefits, which also increase with the child's age and special needs and may include respite care and clothing allowances. Grandparents may receive foster care benefits for a grandchild, but only if that child is a dependent of the juvenile court system and meets selected criteria (see "Foster Care Assistance," below). This means that of the children who are abused and abandoned by their parents and living with relatives, only those placed by court order may be eligible for the higher benefits.

One couple in Missouri took in five grandchildren when their son and daughter-in-law lost custody. Each month they receive less than $388 in welfare benefits for the care and feeding of five growing children. "We are now behind in our bills," he writes. "Our utilities are about to get cut off, and we can't seem to make ends meet. We don't want to send these children to a foster home, but with these financial problems, we are almost forced to send them to one." Had these children qualified for foster care, the family would have received at least $1,355 a month, an average of $271 per child.[1] To quote one grandmother in Cleveland, "No one can tell you you're raising your grandchild for money!"

Social Stigma

Perhaps the hardest thing about asking for help is the social stigma. Too many people think welfare is synonymous with being lazy instead of needy, and that attitude can be reflected by many state and county employees. Grandparents often receive scorn rather than sympathy when they take in a grandchild and need to seek aid. Some grandparents don't look like they need assistance and are made to feel guilty about asking for it. There are eligibility workers who act as if they're pulling money out of their own pockets. "You do walk on eggshells when you deal with social services," says Ada MacKenzie. "Those people talk to you like they talk to a dog."

Grandparents who get foster care benefits have it slightly easier. They don't have to sit in line at the welfare office to talk to eligibility workers. Because they are taking over for the state, they are treated more like Good Samaritans than welfare recipients—although the only difference between the two might be a call to child protective services.

This kind of prejudice, like bureaucracy, is a frustrating reality of government assistance. You can try to ignore it. You can air out your feelings in a support group or with other grandparents. But try not to let it eat away at you; it will only drain you of the energy you need to raise your grandchildren. The truth is, every grandparent who takes in a child is doing something wonderful for society. If these kids went to the state, the state would be putting out a lot more money and resources to care for them.

Don't be discouraged. These programs exist to help children in need. If your grandchildren qualify for them, they deserve the assistance. And you deserve the financial relief. Even if what you get from welfare isn't enough to raise a child, it still helps, and every bit of help counts. A few hundred dollars can make a great difference to a grandparent struggling on a fixed income, and the medical assistance can be a lifesaver if you cannot put your grandchildren on your insurance policy.

The rest of this chapter looks at federal assistance programs one by one. It discusses what they are, what you get, what you need to qualify for them, and what you as a grandparent need to know to receive the most help. Each program description is only a blueprint of what you may encounter. Although these are federally sponsored programs, they are administered by state, county, and local governments, and their regulations and benefits often vary. Also, many of these programs are subject to change whenever welfare and health care reforms take effect. So, consider this chapter a primer; it offers enough information to spark questions. Then check local resources for current, detailed information about the implementation of federal assistance programs in your state. Remember, the more information you have, the better armed you are to work the system—instead of being worked over by the system.

WELFARE ASSISTANCE

What It Is

Welfare assistance is a government program designed to provide needy children and their caregivers with monthly cash assistance to help pay for basic needs like food, clothing, and rent. For almost 60 years, the major source of welfare assistance in the United States was a federal program known as AFDC (Aid to Families with Dependent Children). The federal government set general guidelines for AFDC, and each state set its own definition of neediness, established its own income limits and benefit levels, and administered the program. In 1996, federal welfare reform eliminated AFDC and created a new program, TANF (Temporary Assistance for Needy Families), which gives states greater freedom in deciding who will get aid, what they will receive, and for how long. In effect, it enables each state to design its own welfare program, within certain parameters.

It is important to know both terms—AFDC and TANF—because while TANF effectively eliminated AFDC, other assistance programs still reference pre-reform AFDC guidelines, and you may still hear both terms mentioned. Additionally, each state may assign its own name to TANF. For instance, the California TANF program is called CalWORKs.

Remember, volatile economies, shifting administrations, and the push for more reforms will continue to alter the welfare landscape. Consider this discussion a general blueprint for assistance, a tool to help you ask questions about the rules and regulations in your own state and county.

Who Is Eligible

In order to qualify for welfare a child must fulfill three major requirements: He must be (1) deprived of parental support, (2) living with a relative caregiver, and (3) poor or financially needy. In most instances, if you are raising your grandchild, he is eligible for welfare benefits. But let's look at the requirements one at a time:

Deprived of Parental Support

The government considers children deprived, or dependent, if they are living without the support of at least one parent because that parent is dead, absent, disabled, unemployed, or "underemployed." Most children who live with their grandparents are deprived of parental support, but they must have been eligible for welfare while living with their parent(s).

Living with a Relative Caregiver

If you are a grandparent and your grandchild is living in your home, you are, by definition, a relative caregiver.

Poor or Financially Needy

In order to be financially eligible for welfare, the income and resources of the child's "assistance unit" must be below certain federal and state limits. An assistance unit is basically the parent(s) of a dependent child, the child, and any dependent brothers or sisters in the home.

Only the income of the child, the parents, and the siblings can be used to determine financial need and only if they live in the same house. The income of parents who do not live with or help support a child does not count toward the child's welfare grant (although the government may go after the parents for reimbursement or child support). Nor should your income affect your grandchild's application. Unless your grandchildren have their own regular source of income, they will probably qualify as needy.

Relative caregivers, even guardians, have no legal responsibility to financially support a child. In most states, your finances should not be considered. The exception is if you yourself are in financial need and want to apply for aid *with* your grandchild; in that case, your income and resources will be taken into consideration (although your home, furniture, and most personal possessions will not be).

Miscellaneous Requirements

There are also several additional requirements your grandchild must satisfy before she can receive welfare assistance. The child must be a U.S. citizen or qualified immigrant* and a legal resident of your state. She must also be under 18 (under 19 if a full-time student) and have a valid Social Security number. If there are any other rules that apply to your family, your grandchild's caseworker should be able to explain them to you.

---

*The government has several definitions of "qualified immigrant." Ask at the welfare office.

What You Get

Welfare assistance typically means monthly cash benefits, or a mix of cash, vouchers, and services. Some recipients may also be eligible for medical assistance and, occasionally, food stamps. The amount of money a family can receive depends on the number of people in the family unit and on the amount and source of income. Benefits vary from state to state and sometimes from county to county. For example, in 2009 a two-person family (presumably parent and child) on welfare could have received a maximum of $162 a month in Arkansas, $355 in Ohio, $561 in California, and as much as $821 in Alaska. The national median that year was $344 for a family of two.[2]

Medical assistance is another possible benefit with welfare. Although the programs are no longer linked, many families receiving welfare assistance are also eligible for Medicaid or their state's equivalent. Additionally, many children who don't qualify for welfare may still qualify for Medicaid; make sure you ask about it for your grandchild. (See "Medicaid," later in this chapter.)

Many welfare families are also eligible to receive supplemental nutritional assistance, commonly known as food stamps. While a grandparent's income may not be considered for welfare eligibility, it will be counted for food stamps. Thus, it is possible that you could receive welfare for your grandchildren but not qualify for food stamps. Even so, it is worth a try. (See "Supplemental Nutritional Assistance Program [SNAP]," later in this chapter.)

The Application Process

How It Should Work

You can apply for welfare assistance at your state or local welfare office. Call ahead to confirm office hours and make sure you have the right office for your area. Find out if you need an appointment or if you can just come in. (See "What You Need to Bring," below.)

To apply for welfare assistance you must file a written application and pass income and resources tests. The welfare office has a responsibility to help you with your application and to help you get the documentation you need. My experience has been that they don't often do this, but they should. If you run into problems, contact your Legal Aid office.

Your application should be processed within 45 days. If aid is denied, the denial must be in writing. If you feel this decision was unfair, you can request a "fair hearing." The written denial usually has to explain how to do this.

Once you begin to receive welfare assistance, you must make monthly reports about your grandchild's income (and about yours, if you applied with your grandchild). The amount of the benefits will be determined month to month, based on each month's circumstances. You will also face a periodic "redetermination," a process in which the welfare department reviews each family's eligibility as if it were a new application.

What You Need to Bring

When you go for your intake interview, try to take as many records as possible to prove your grandchild's eligibility (and yours, if you are applying with your grandchild). Make sure you have photocopies for the application. Never give away your originals. Don't panic if you can't put your hands on everything; it is the responsibility of the welfare office to reasonably help you get all the required documentation.

To apply for welfare for your grandchild, you will need the following:

- Proof of the child's age and identity, for example, a birth certificate (few grandparents actually have their grandchild's birth certificate, but you can request a copy from the county where your grandchild was born).
- Proof of the child's residence, for example, school records or a letter to the address.
- The child's Social Security number.
- Proof of your tie to the child (the parent's birth certificate, along with the child's birth certificate, should establish your relationship).
- Proof of income of the child (if any).
- Proof of the child's citizenship or immigration status.

The welfare office cannot limit you to a particular form of identification or proof. For instance, if you cannot find a birth certificate, you should be able to use another proof of age or identity. Even an affidavit might be sufficient while other forms of proof are sought.

■ WHAT YOU NEED TO KNOW

• *You will need to ask lots of questions and double-check answers.* There is great confusion out there about how grandparents apply for aid for their grandchildren and how aid is determined. Many eligibility workers are used to dealing with regular parent–child applications. They may not know how the laws and regulations affect grandparents, and they often give out information that is simply wrong. It's not uncommon for social workers to call GAP for help with resources and have no idea that there is a kinship resource center or liaison in their own department. That's how much kinship is still under the radar. Keep asking. Ask various people. Ask more than once. If your grandchild is eligible for assistance, don't let misinformation deprive him of it.

• *Your income should not count.* One of the biggest problems a grandparent faces with a welfare application is answering the questions about income. These are equally baffling to eligibility workers, who consistently give out the wrong information and often count Grandma's income when they shouldn't.

Unless you are applying for assistance *with* your grandchild, or you have adopted your grandchild, your income should not count in most states. You should be considered a "non-needy caregiver," seeking a "child-only" grant. This means you are filling out that application for your grandchild, not for yourself. Despite what they tell you, fill out the form *as if you were the child.* For instance: If the question is "Do you own a home?" the answer is no (you may own a home, but the child does not). If the question is "Do you have a bank account?," the answer is no if the child does not have a bank account. It shouldn't matter what your income and circumstances are; if your state offers child-only grants, your grandchild should be eligible for assistance. This is true even if you become a legal guardian. If you fill out the forms based on *your* income, the application will be denied. That is exactly what happened to Janet Baker when she was given the wrong information at the welfare office. Not only did they turn her down, but they made her feel awful for even daring to ask for help. "It was three months before I finally got some assistance for the children," says Janet. "By that time, our financial situation was even worse. I felt really battered. The process of finding out just how to do that was a major step for me."

Although federal guidelines no longer require states to provide child-only grants, most states still offer them. Double-check with several sources before taking no for an answer.

- *You can apply for welfare for yourself.* If you are raising a welfare-eligible child and you yourself meet the criteria for welfare benefits, you may apply with your grandchild as an assistance unit. Even if your grandchild receives Supplemental Security Income (SSI) or foster care benefits (see below), he may still qualify your family for welfare, although he won't count toward the amount of assistance you receive.[3] Be advised that federal TANF guidelines impose a lifetime maximum limit of five years for adults who receive assistance; they also include work requirements. However, there may also be additional state-funded programs that are not as restrictive.

- *You should keep records.* Papers get lost and conversations forgotten. Remember to keep copies of all the documents you turn in to any welfare office. Also, keep track of all conversations you have and all attempted contacts with agency personnel. If you can, send letters that confirm any information you receive, and keep copies of those letters. If your information is incorrect, the agency should write back and correct it. If not, you have it confirmed in writing. This could be useful if you ever have to appeal.

- *You can appeal.* If your application is denied or your benefits are discontinued, you must be notified in writing. If you feel that your benefits have been denied or discontinued unfairly or that you are not receiving the correct amount of aid or that you are being mistreated by a welfare worker, you have the right to request a state hearing. Although this can be done by filling out a hearing request form or making a phone call, the most efficient way to request a hearing is to fill out the form on the back of your denial notice. Photocopy both sides of the notice for your records before you return it.

- *You may want to get legal representation.* If you do appeal, it can be helpful to have an advocate or an attorney handle your case. Grandparents who cannot afford counsel can sometimes find pro bono or discounted help through organizations like Legal Aid or welfare rights groups. The Legal Aid Foundation of Los Angeles has helped some of our grandparents appeal government decisions and receive aid they could not get on their own.

FOSTER CARE ASSISTANCE

What It Is

Foster care benefits—properly known as federal Title IV-E (four-E) foster care—are a type of assistance benefits for children who have been removed from their homes by CPS and are living somewhere else.[4] Federal foster care may also be available in cases where a child has been placed with a relative. Some areas may also have state and county foster care programs, which may not apply to relatives.

Who Is Eligible

For your grandchild to qualify for federal foster care, she must fulfill three general requirements: she must be (1) a dependent of the court, (2) AFDC-eligible and AFDC-linked, and (3) in an approved placement. These requirements get confusing, particularly since states vary on their interpretations of the law, so let's look at them one at a time:

Dependent of the Court

To be a dependent of the court your grandchild must have been removed from her parents, other relatives, or legal guardian and placed with you by a juvenile court order or a voluntary placement agreement with CPS. If you have taken your grandchild into your home or if CPS placed the child with you without a court order, she will not be eligible for foster care benefits.

AFDC-Eligible and AFDC-Linked

Foster care still references the old AFDC program to determine federal eligibility. For foster care, AFDC-eligible simply means that your grandchild fulfills the major pre–welfare reform requirements for AFDC eligibility—

that is, he is deprived of parental support, needy (by former AFDC standards), and living with a relative—as well as the additional requirements of age, residence, and a Social Security number.

AFDC-linked is more complicated. This is the requirement that is most open to interpretation and confusion. According to federal law, AFDC linkage means any one of the following three things:

1. The child was receiving AFDC in the home from which he was removed in the month the child welfare agency petitioned for his removal, *or*
2. The child could have received AFDC in that home if the parent had applied in the month of the court petition, *or*
3. The child was living in the home from which he was removed within the six months before the petition was filed and could have received AFDC in that home (that is, with the parent).

The question of whether a child *could have* received AFDC centers on the child's financial situation in the month he was removed. If the child was removed from his parent's home, the parent's income counts toward AFDC eligibility. The difficulty with this requirement is that in order to determine if the child was eligible you often need to talk to the parent who had custody if you need information about the parent's finances. Unfortunately, the parent may not be around or may be too angry or too high to be helpful. If the parent is available and cooperative, getting this information is not a problem. If the parent was receiving welfare at that time, it is also not a problem, since the welfare office has access to those records. But if he or she is missing or uncooperative, you could have a tough time meeting this requirement. (Note: It is the child services agency's responsibility to establish the parent[s]' income for purposes of meeting this requirement. However, as a relative, if you have information that could be helpful to determine the parent's income, it is important to provide it to the social worker.)

Another problem with linkage is that while federal law says one thing, states often pass regulations that say something else, sometimes creating policies that are more restrictive than federal requirements. This means that children who are eligible for family foster care funding under federal law could still be denied federal benefits because of individual state regulations. If your grandchild meets your state requirements for AFDC linkage, you don't have a problem. If he doesn't meet state requirements but meets federal requirements, you can request a fair hearing.

Approved Placement

The last requirement for federal foster care assistance is that the child be in an approved placement. That means the child is placed in the home of a relative approved by the child welfare agency or in a licensed foster care facility.

What You Get

Foster care benefits include monthly cash benefits, health care services through Medicaid, and some additional social services. Foster care benefits are higher than welfare benefits because foster children are presumed to have greater needs than children on welfare. Unlike welfare, where benefits are determined by family size, foster care is based on the age and needs of each child. In many areas, special needs children—those who are developmentally delayed, physically challenged, prenatally drug exposed, and so on—may also be entitled to additional benefits called "specialized care rates." These rates increase the amount of a child's foster care grant. However, states and counties vary regarding the specialized rates they provide and the eligibility requirements for them. If you think your grandchild qualifies for specialized care rates, talk to the social worker. If the child qualifies, you may be required to attend a short training course about handling those special needs.

Foster children automatically qualify for Medicaid and may also be eligible for certain social services, including a clothing allowance, free school breakfast and lunch, and, occasionally, respite care. However, both the dollar amount of foster care benefits and the scope of health care coverage and services vary state by state, and sometimes even within individual states.

Foster care benefits typically continue until a child's 18th birthday or until he graduates from high school or turns 19, whichever comes first. However, in some states, foster care benefits can extend until the child is 21 as long as the child remains in an approved foster care placement (including supervised independent living), continues his education or job training, or works at least part time.[5]

Although foster care benefits only address the needs of the dependent child, you may be able to apply for welfare assistance for yourself while you receive foster care benefits for your grandchild if you are financially needy.

The Application Process

How It Should Work

The children's services worker should be the one to start the application process for you. Once the child has been removed by child protection and placed with you by court order or, in some circumstances, a formal voluntary placement agreement with CPS, the children's services worker is supposed to explain your benefit choices, which in most cases consist of either welfare assistance or foster care assistance (if the child qualifies).

For many grandparents, choosing between welfare and family foster care benefits can be something of a gamble. It is easier to qualify for welfare assistance, but foster care benefits are higher. If you go with welfare but your grandchild was eligible for foster care, you lose the higher benefits. On the other hand, if you choose foster care and a month later discover that your grandchild doesn't qualify, you will have lost a month of welfare benefits. You can apply for welfare assistance while you are waiting for a foster care decision (see "What You Need to Know," below).

Once you decide, the worker should either help you collect the information you need to establish the child's eligibility for foster care benefits or, if you choose welfare assistance, process your grandchild's welfare application. He should also explain your foster care rights and responsibilities and immediately obtain a Medicaid card for your grandchild.

How It Often Works

Unfortunately, social workers often neglect to explain government benefits to relative caregivers. I have had grandparents call me months, and even years, after a child was placed with them by the court, and they hadn't even known the child was eligible for benefits and Medicaid.

■ WHAT YOU NEED TO KNOW

• *Federal foster care is a court-related program.* To be eligible for federal foster care benefits, your grandchildren must be placed in your home by a court order or voluntary placement agreement with CPS. If the parents just leave them with you or if you take them in informally, they will not be eligible for these benefits: Say, for example, your granddaughter calls and tells you that Mom has been sleeping for two days and there is no food in the house. If you simply pick her up and never involve the courts, she will not qualify for foster care. If, on the other hand, you call a social worker and make a referral of neglect *and* if CPS removes the child *and* if Mom would have been eligible for AFDC and signs the necessary papers, or was already receiving it, then the child should be eligible for federal foster care benefits.

The problem is that most grandparents won't leave children in a neglectful situation in the hopes that a social worker will get there in time. They will rush in to rescue their grandchildren—and end up paying for it in the pocket. Foster care is related to court placement, and the courts only get involved when a child is in danger. If you have the child and the parent is not an immediate threat to her safety, the child welfare system may consider the child well protected and refuse to open a case. One social worker told a grandmother that the only way to become a foster parent would be to abandon her grandchildren, have them placed in foster care, and then apply for custody. Of course, Grandma knew that there was no guarantee she would actually get the children and that in the meantime they ran the risk of being further traumatized. Grandma stayed with lower benefits.[6]

• *Voluntary placement agreements are time-limited.* If your grandchild comes to you via a voluntary placement agreement, be aware that it lasts a maximum of six months. If the child is not returned to the parent before the expiration date, CPS must file a removal petition with the court.

• *You can apply for welfare and foster care assistance at the same time.* Relatives are sometimes told they can apply for either welfare or foster care, but not both. They are also told that once they make a choice and benefits start, they cannot change their minds. Neither of these statements is true. While you cannot receive duplicate aid for the same child in the same period, nothing in the law prevents you from applying for both, especially if there is a chance that the child might not qualify for federal foster care assistance. You can also start on welfare and then switch to foster care if your grandchild qualifies.

If you apply only for foster care and are approved, your grandchild will receive the higher rate dating back to the day that your home was approved. If, instead, you also apply for and receive welfare while you wait for foster care approval, the welfare payments will be deducted from the retroactive benefits. However, if you apply only for foster care assistance and are eventually denied, your grandchild will have gone several months without any benefits at all. This is particularly hard on lower-income grandparents who not only need the higher benefits but also need immediate help.

• *You can appeal.* If your grandchild does not qualify for foster care benefits and if you dispute that decision, you can request a state fair hearing.

SUPPLEMENTAL SECURITY INCOME (SSI) FOR CHILDREN

What It Is

Like welfare assistance, SSI is a federal cash assistance program for people in need. But while welfare is designed to help children who are poor and deprived, SSI assists those who are poor and blind or disabled. Also, SSI typically offers higher benefits than welfare and does not automatically end at 18. At age 18, children who continue to meet SSI financial requirements are reevaluated based on the adult standards and may continue to receive benefits if they still qualify as disabled.

Who Is Eligible

Three factors determine SSI eligibility for children under 18: financial need, disability, and immigration status. Your grandchild must fill all requirements to qualify for SSI benefits.

Financial Need

Financial need is based on the income and assets of the child, not the guardian. Your financial situation should not affect your grandchild's application. However, SSI will count any welfare, foster care, or adoption assistance benefits your grandchild receives, as well as Social Security Survivors Benefits (see below). Each state sets its own eligibility limits, within federal guidelines, for income and resources.

Disability

For SSI purposes, children are considered disabled if they have a physical or mental condition that results in marked and severe functional limitations. In other words, the condition keeps them from doing things and behaving in ways that are normal for other children of the same age. This disability must also be one that is expected to last at least 12 months or result in the child's death. Federal law and Social Security regulations include a specific list of conditions that qualify as disabilities. If your grandchild's condition is not on that list, he may still be found eligible if his condition, or combination of conditions, meets a condition on the list.

Immigration Status

To be eligible for SSI, your grandchild must be a citizen of the United States or a legal resident as of August 22, 1996. If your grandchild established legal residency after that date, contact your local SSA office to determine his eligibility.

What You Get

In most states, children who qualify for SSI receive cash assistance, as well as health care services through Medicaid and the Children with Special Health Care Needs (CSHCN) program.

Monthly Cash Benefits

How much cash assistance your grandchild receives depends on where you live, since many states supplement the federal program with state funding.

Health Care Services

In addition to Medicaid, SSI children are usually entitled to additional health care services under the Children with Special Health Care Needs (CSHCN) provisions of the Social Security Act. CSHCN programs are usually administered by state health agencies. The names and regulations of these programs vary from state to state, but most offer specialized services through private doctors, clinics, hospitals, and community agencies. A child who is not eligible for cash assistance through SSI may still be eligible for medical assistance through a local CSHCN program. Check with your local health department, social services office, or hospital for more information.

The Application Process

How It Should Work

You can apply for SSI by calling the Social Security Administration (SSA) and scheduling an interview with your local Social Security office. You will need to fill out an application for SSI, which can be completed by telephone or in person, and a Child Disability Report, which can be completed in person, by phone, or online.

Once you apply, the local Social Security office will decide whether your grandchild's income and assets/resources are within federal and state SSI limits. Then all the information about your grandchild's medical condition will be sent to a state agency, usually called the Disability Determination Service (DDS), for review by doctors and other trained staff. The DDS team will look at how your grandchild's condition affects her functioning in everyday life to decide if she meets the SSI criteria for disability. To do this, they will consider both medical and nonmedical evidence (that is, letters from teachers, doctors, child care providers, etc.). If your grandchild does not have thorough medical records, you may be asked to take the child for a special exam that Social Security will pay for,[7] but it is better to have reports from his own doctors. You will also face a periodic "redetermination," a process in which the SSA department reviews your grandchild's income, resources, and living arrangements to make sure he is still eligible for, and getting the right amount of, SSI benefits.

How It Often Works

It is not uncommon for the SSA to take more than six months to decide SSI eligibility, and even then many cases are incorrectly denied, often owing to a lack of medical or psychiatric documentation. However, many denials are overturned on appeal. If your grandchild is denied, you have a legal right to appeal the decision. If the appeal is successful, he may even receive retroactive benefits based upon the date of the original application.

What You Need to Bring

The more information you bring to your SSI appointment, the easier it will be for Social Security to process your grandchild's application. You will need two kinds of documentation for your grandchild's SSI application: records that show income eligibility and those that confirm the child's disability.

To show your grandchild's income eligibility, you will need to bring the child's

- Social Security number
- Birth certificate or other proof of age
- Financial records and other information about the child's income and resources
- Proof of citizenship or immigration status (birth certificate, green card, visa, passport, immigration papers, etc.)

To prove your grandchild's disability, you must describe, in as much detail as possible, how the disability prevents him from doing things that other children of the same age can normally do. Just because a child is born drug exposed, for instance, is not enough to qualify him as disabled. While some children are indeed severely disabled from prenatal drug exposure, others seem to function normally. DDS needs thorough, detailed information. Records that can help include:

- *Medical records.* Bring information on *all* medical problems, past and present, that the child has experienced, including a list of all his medications. Even problems that seem unrelated to the disability could be important. In fact, to avoid forgetting anything in the interview, you might consider making a list of all the reasons you think your grandchild is disabled.

• *List of medical personnel.* Bring the names, addresses, and phone numbers of all doctors, hospitals, clinics, and specialists who have treated the child. Be as specific as possible. If you can, provide dates of visits and medical account numbers to help get records as soon as possible.

• *Nonmedical records.* Social Security doesn't just use medical evidence to decide a child's eligibility for SSI. The agency also considers evidence that shows whether a child can do "age-appropriate activities." Since the disability examiner is not able to see the child, he has to rely on reports from nonmedical sources about what the child can and cannot do and how she manages everyday tasks. Helpful nonmedical records include school records; special education or early intervention plans, if the child has one (see Chapter 13); and the names and addresses of teachers, therapists, social workers, child care providers, clergy, relatives, and neighbors who can describe the child's ability to perform everyday activities.

• *Letters with specific examples.* If possible, ask all your medical and nonmedical sources to provide you with written reports about your grandchild in addition to their standard records. Ask them—as well as family members and clergy—to describe in detail how the disability interferes with the child's everyday activities and to give specific examples. Write down your own observations about your grandchild's disability as well.

Don't wait to have all your paperwork together before you apply. Although it can take months to decide whether your grandchild qualifies for SSI, the payments will go back to the date of your initial visit or phone call as long as the application is filed within the following 60 days. The Social Security staff is supposed to help you find missing documents or suggest substitutes, and many communities have special arrangements between medical providers, social service agencies, and schools.

■ WHAT YOU NEED TO KNOW

• *You don't have to mail original documents.* Although the SSA requires original documents to process your application, you can take them in to your local Social Security office in person and they can make the copies they need and immediately return your originals.

• *It's important to get things in writing.* When government workers tell you anything about your case—whether they are giving you instructions or notifying you of changes—ask them to put it in writing. Also, keep copies of anything you send to government offices. On the copy, mark the date you mailed the letter and, if you can, send it certified so you can verify that Social Security got it.

• *Your grandchild's doctor can do the evaluation.* SSI decides most cases on the basis of medical assessments. A child has a right to have evidence submitted by her own doctor and to have that individual conduct the follow-up assessments as well. If there is a need for additional testing, Social Security should pay for it, whether the agency uses your grandchild's physician or its own.[8]

• *There are special cases.* Although Social Security can take several months to evaluate whether a child is disabled, there are exceptions. Individuals whose condition is so severe that they are automatically presumed to be disabled can receive SSI benefits for up to six months while the formal disability decision is being made. These conditions include, but are not limited to, HIV infection; blindness; Down syndrome; and some cases of deafness, cerebral palsy, and muscular dystrophy.[9]

• *Immigrants may have other options.* Although SSI is available only to U.S. citizens and legal residents, some states have state-funded programs to help immigrants who are aged, blind, or disabled. For instance, California has a program called CAPI (Cash Assistance Program for Immigrants), which provides benefits to those who meet all SSI criteria except immigration status. If your grandchild falls into that category, ask your welfare office if your state has anything similar.

• *Cash gifts to your grandchild will count against the SSI benefits.* If you want to give the child a gift or start a college fund, set up a "blocked trust" account that he or she cannot access; otherwise, it may count as income.

• *SSA must be notified about changes.* Once your grandchild gets SSI, you must notify the SSA about any change in his address, income, medical condition, living arrangements, and school attendance. The agency must be notified if he leaves the United States. If you do not report these changes on time, your grandchild could lose his SSI eligibility.

- *It is important to keep receipts.* SSI is only for the daily support of the eligible child, and you must account for this money every year.
- *SSA deposits SSI checks electronically to your bank.* If at all possible, you should also keep these funds in a separate account. However, it is still important to keep detailed records of how this money is spent.
- *During the appeal process, your grandchild may still be eligible for welfare assistance and Medicaid.* Appealing an SSI denial can be a long process, and you won't receive benefits for your grandchild during the course of it. If you do appeal an SSI denial, see if you can apply for welfare and Medicaid in the meantime.
- *You may want to get legal assistance.* The appeal process can be long and complicated. It can be helpful to have an attorney or advocate in your camp. If you can't afford an attorney, your local Legal Aid office may be able to help you. If your grandchild is developmentally delayed or mentally ill, you may be able to get legal assistance through a Protection and Advocacy office in your state (see Appendix A, Parenting and Education Resources, National Disability Rights Network). Some private attorneys also take selected cases on a contingency fee, meaning that they get paid only if you win your appeal. Talk to your state or local bar association for referrals.

SOCIAL SECURITY SURVIVORS BENEFITS

What It Is

Social Security Survivors Benefits are monthly insurance payments to children under 18 who have a deceased parent. When most people think of Social Security, they think of retirement benefits, but Social Security taxes also pay into survivors' insurance for certain family members, including minor children.

Who Is Eligible

To be eligible for Social Security Survivors Benefits, a child must be under 18 (full-time students under 19 and older disabled children are also eligible), unmarried, and the dependent of a parent who has died. The parent in question must have worked, paid Social Security taxes, and earned enough credits to generate benefits. Because my sister didn't earn enough Social Security credits before she died, my nephew Kevin wasn't eligible for Survivors Benefits; he received only welfare assistance and Medicaid.

A child's disability is not relevant for Social Security Survivors Benefits; only the parent's work history is. According to the Social Security Administration, 98 percent of children are eligible for benefits if a working parent should die.[10]

What You Get

Children who qualify for Social Security Survivors Benefits receive monthly cash benefits. These benefits are based on the average lifetime earnings of the parent and on how much the parent paid into Social Security while he or she worked. A child can receive both SSI and Survivors Benefits if she is eligible for both based on income and other requirements.

The Application Process
How It Should Work

Apply promptly by phone or at any Social Security office since. According to the SSA, a child's claim for survivor's benefits can be retroactive to the month of death, but only within six months. And, in some cases, benefits may only be retroactive to the date of application. Even if you don't have all your paperwork together, apply anyway. The Social Security office should help you collect any documentation you need.

What You Need to Bring

You will need original documents or certified copies of the child's Social Security card and birth certificate, the parent's Social Security number, the parent's death certificate, and the deceased parent's W-2 forms or federal tax return (if self-employed) for the most recent year. You should also bring a checkbook or savings passbook, as benefits are deposited electronically to an account each month.

ADOPTION ASSISTANCE PROGRAM (AAP)

What It Is

Adoption assistance (sometimes "adoption subsidy") is a federal assistance program—administered through the states—that provides monthly benefits and other services to children whose adoption may depend on financial aid. States also have programs for children who may not be eligible for federal adoption assistance.

Foster children are eligible for financial, social, and medical assistance, including Medicaid, all of which they typically lose when they are adopted. Most adoptive parents willingly shoulder the financial responsibility for these children in exchange for the security of adoption. With respect to some children, however, there are circumstances that place added burdens on their caregivers: They may suffer from a physical disability or an emotional disorder, or they may be part of a sibling group that must be placed together. Relatives or foster parents who care for these children may depend on the government assistance they receive; it may be that they simply cannot afford to adopt the child without it. AAP is designed to provide financial assistance to encourage the adoption of these "special needs" children.

Adoption assistance lasts until the child is 18 years old. It can be discontinued earlier if the adoptive parent is no longer legally responsible and financially supporting the child, and states may extend eligibility to age 21 if the child is physically or mentally disabled. This extension is not automatic, however, and must be requested before the child turns 18.

Who Is Eligible

Special needs children are children who have situations or conditions that make it difficult to find an adoptive home for them without assistance. These might include age, race, or ethnicity; a background of severe neglect or abuse; inclusion in a sibling group; a family history of mental illness; or a disability (physical, medical, mental, or emotional). The situations and conditions that constitute "special needs" vary from state to state. While AAP is partially funded by the federal government, each state defines its own eligibility requirements.

Before he can be considered a special needs child, the state must verify that a child cannot or should not be returned to his family, that he is free for adoption, and that reasonable efforts have been made to place him in a family without financial aid.

There are also eligibility requirements for adoption assistance, which serves children who would have received federal assistance if they had not been adopted. Therefore, federal AAP benefits are available only to children who (1) are getting federal foster care payments at the time of adoption, (2) are receiving SSI at the time of adoption, (3) have been in foster care for five or more consecutive years, or (4) are age 10 or older by September 30, 2013. This age limit will drop yearly (by two years of age) until 2018, at which point all children who exit foster care will be eligible for AAP, provided the court properly determined that the child could not be returned to his or her parents.

As with welfare assistance, your income will not affect your grandchild's eligibility for federal AAP, although it may affect the amount of monthly aid he receives.

What You Get

Children who are eligible receive monthly cash payments, medical assistance, and, occasionally, additional help, such as respite care, specialized day care, counseling, and other social services that might be provided to foster parents. Adoptive parents may also be eligible for reimbursement for one-time, or "nonrecurring," adoption expenses, which may include adoption fees, court costs, and attorney fees.

Adoption assistance benefits are negotiated between the administering agency and your family and are based on your financial circumstances and the particular needs of the child you are adopting. Actual rates vary from state to state, but they cannot be more than the family foster care benefits for which your grandchild would be eligible.

Children who qualify for the federal program automatically receive Medicaid. Medicaid coverage varies from state to state, and most states cover children who are not federally eligible, although some require that the child have a disability that warrants Medicaid.

The Application Process

How It Should Work

The Adoption Assistance Agreement is a legal document that is negotiated between the adoptive parent and the state or county adoption agency. Each agreement is based on the needs of the particular child. The agreement specifies the amount of the payments; the eligibility requirements for Medicaid and social services; and the other payments, services, and assistance programs that are available. The agreement includes wording that guarantees that it will be in effect regardless of what state you live in, and it includes provisions to protect the child's interests if you move to a new state.

You can apply for adoption assistance when you begin the adoption process for your grandchild. Sometimes an adoption worker will deliver a proposed Adoption Assistance Agreement when she comes to assess your home. Otherwise, make sure you ask about it. Once you do apply, look at the initial agreement carefully. If it is not acceptable, negotiate it *before* the adoption goes through. The benefit rate should not be lower than any foster care benefits you have been receiving. Afterward, you must report any change in your family circumstances, and you may need to recertify the agreement on a regular basis, depending on your state. (See the link to the Adoption Assistance by State Database in the Child Welfare Information Gateway section of Appendix A for state-specific information.)

■ WHAT YOU NEED TO KNOW

- *Adoption assistance isn't a favor.* If your grandchild qualifies for adoption assistance, he is entitled to it. Find out what your state's criteria for AAP are, and don't be afraid to ask.
- *Previously adopted children still count.* If you are adopting a previously adopted child—perhaps one who was being raised by another grandparent or your child who died—and she is already receiving federal AAP, eligibility does not need to be reestablished. You will, however, have to apply in your state of residence.
- *Children of teen parents may be eligible.* If you are adopting a grandchild who is a teen parent and exiting foster care, ask about AAP for both the parent and child.

• *Negotiation should precede adoption.* Negotiate and sign the adoption assistance agreement before you adopt your grandchild. Once the adoption is final, the state has no incentive to negotiate with you.

• *Even negotiation for AAP benefits for at-risk children should precede adoption.* Think ahead. Your grandchild may not appear to have serious problems, but certain circumstances like prenatal drug exposure or a mentally ill parent could make her vulnerable to problems in the future. According to policy advocate Josh Kroll, if you have reason to believe that your grandchild is at risk for future problems, some states allow you to still apply for AAP benefits; the agreement you sign will say that your grandchild does not qualify for cash assistance now but that her eligibility can be addressed again if problems arise in the future.[11] However, you must negotiate this agreement and complete the paperwork before you adopt your grandchild.

• *Ask about the federal adoption tax credit.* The adoption tax credit is a federal tax credit designed to encourage adoption and is calculated per child. Even if you receive AAP and didn't pay any adoption expenses for your grandchild, it's worth asking about the tax credit.[12]

• *It's a good idea to talk to a legal expert.* An attorney or an advocate who is familiar with adoption assistance can help you understand the various services and assistance to which your grandchild may be entitled. He can also identify which services are most important to the child, negotiate modifications of the agreement, enforce the agreement, or appeal decisions. If you have an attorney handling your adoption, talk to him about AAP. If not, consider talking to someone. I know a grandmother in Pittsburgh who adopted her grandchild. When she asked about assistance, the social worker asked her why she wasn't happy enough to get her grandchild and why she needed to apply for money, too. Sometimes it's easier to have a professional handle these issues for you.

KINSHIP GUARDIANSHIP ASSISTANCE PROGRAM

What It Is

The Kinship Guardianship Assistance Program (called KinGAP in some states) is a federal cash assistance program that provides monthly benefits for children who are exiting the foster care system into a permanent placement with a relative guardian who is unable or unwilling to adopt.

Foster children are eligible for financial, social, and medical assistance, including Medicaid. Relatives who care for these children may depend on the government assistance they receive and may not be able to afford to create a permanent plan without it.

KinGAP assistance lasts until the child is 18, or in some cases 21, provided the guardian remains legally responsible for the child and continues to support her. It can be discontinued earlier if the legal guardian is no longer legally responsible for the support of the child.

Who Is Eligible

Kinship guardianship assistance programs are funded by the federal government, but each state defines its own eligibility requirements, and some states offer their own subsidized guardianship assistance. Generally, however, a child is eligible for KinGAP if returning home and adoption have both been ruled out as permanency options and the following criteria are met:

- He has lived with the prospective relative guardian for at least six months while eligible for federal foster care benefits, whether or not he received them (see above).
- He demonstrates a strong attachment to—and a stable, ongoing relationship with—the prospective relative guardian.
- If he is 14 or older, he agrees to the guardianship arrangement.

Some states also extend eligibility to the sibling of an eligible child, even if she herself does not fit the criteria, provided they are placed together.

A prospective relative guardian is eligible for KinGAP if the following criteria are met:

- She is unwilling or unable to adopt but demonstrates a strong commitment to caring for the child on a permanent basis.
- She has been identified as the best permanent plan for the child.
- All the adults in the household have been screened for criminal and child abuse records.

Some states also require a prospective relative guardian to be a licensed foster parent.

What You Get

Children who are eligible receive monthly cash payments, medical assistance, and, occasionally, additional social services. Children who qualify for the federal program automatically receive Medicaid. Medicaid coverage varies from state to state, and some states cover children who are not federally eligible. KinGAP agreements also include payment for legal services connected to obtaining guardianship (up to $2,000), as well as educational and training vouchers for the child and, in some circumstances, transitional housing.

The Application Process

How It Should Work

The Kinship Guardianship Assistance Agreement is a legally binding guardianship agreement that is negotiated between the prospective relative guardian and the state. Each agreement is based on the needs of the particular child. The agreement specifies the amount of and manner in which the payments will be provided; the eligibility requirements for Medicaid and social services; and the other payments, services, and assistance programs that are available. Federal guardianship assistance is meant to remain in effect regardless of what state you live in,[13] and the agreement should include provisions to protect the child's interests if you move to a new state.

You can ask about kinship guardianship in the permanency planning stage of the dependency process. Make sure to negotiate it *before* filing for guardianship. If you are denied, you may request a fair hearing. The benefit rate should not be lower than any foster care benefits you have been receiving.

■ WHAT YOU NEED TO KNOW

• *Guardianship assistance isn't a favor.* It was designed to help dependent children achieve permanent placement in a stable, loving family. Find out about your state's criteria for KinGAP, and don't be afraid to ask.

• *This is not about special needs.* KinGAP, unlike adoption assistance, does not require a child to have special needs to qualify.

- *Apply separately for siblings.* Each sibling in a sibling group is eligible for her own KinGAP payment and individual reimbursement for nonrecurring legal costs, if such reimbursement is available in your state.

- *KinGAP should move with you.* Kinship guardianship agreements are meant to remain in effect even if you and your grandchildren move to a new state. However this is not always true in every state. Get clear information when you apply.

- *Expect readjustments.* KinGAP payments may be periodically adjusted based on the changing needs of the child and the circumstances of the relative guardian. If a child develops signs of disabilities or special needs, this is an opportunity to request higher benefits.

- *KinGAP doesn't always end at 18.* In some cases, KinGAP payments can extend to 21, provided that the child is still in school (high school, college, or vocational); employed 80 hours a month; participating in a program that promotes or removes barriers to employment; or determined to be incapable of these activities due to a documented medical condition.

HEALTH CARE AND NUTRITION ASSISTANCE

Any parent knows that children run up a small fortune in health care costs. They need vaccinations and school physicals. They get colds, scrapes, and a collection of childhood diseases. The more adventuresome ones sprain and break things as they test their limits and endurance. Moreover, the cost of doctors and medicine is exorbitant. If you add the health risks of prenatal drug exposure or the cost of psychiatric care for traumatized children, your health care costs can run sky high.

Unlike parents, who can get insurance for their children, most grandparents cannot put grandchildren on their insurance policies. A few rare employers have allowed grandkids to be included when a grandparent has guardianship, but most grandparents must adopt their grandchildren in order to get private health insurance for them. This is where government benefits become very important. Even middle-class grandparents, who may be able to support their grandchildren financially, need the medical benefits that are available to their grandchildren.

MEDICAID

What It Is

Medicaid is a health care program for people with low income and limited assets; it helps pay doctor and hospital bills and covers some medications. However, Medicaid is not so much one program as 50 individual programs, with each state providing a different combination of benefits. Although the states all function within the same federal guidelines, there is significant variety in eligibility criteria, as well as in the conditions and treatments covered. What follows is a brief and broad explanation of Medicaid benefits. This information always needs to be confirmed by someone at your state level.

Who Is Eligible

Although Medicaid varies from state to state, children who qualify for federal foster care and SSI automatically qualify for Medicaid. Additionally, many poor children who don't qualify for financial assistance through SSI may still be eligible for Medicaid coverage. Check with your local office to find out if your grandchild is eligible.

What You Get

Medicaid coverage can vary greatly from state to state. However, all participating states must provide children with medically necessary doctor and hospital services, lab work and X-rays, and early screening. In many cases, additional medical services, like prescription drugs, eyeglasses, dental care, counseling, and inpatient psychiatric care for individuals under 21, are also provided. (See "Early Periodic Screening, Diagnosis, and Treatment [EPSDT]," below.)

The Application Process

How It Should Work

In many states Medicaid comes automatically with SSI, welfare, and federal foster care eligibility; the forms might even come together. In other states you will have to sign up for it separately. Be sure to ask. Medicaid coverage is supposed to take effect within 45 days of your application and be retroactive to the day you applied. Additionally, states must provide Medicaid to the child for the three months before the application was filed, if he or she would have been eligible at that time.

How It Often Works

Unfortunately, processing a Medicaid application often takes longer than 45 days, and a medically needy grandchild could exhaust your resources while you wait. Don't let it happen. If you have a problem or an emergency, call your eligibility or welfare worker.

■ WHAT YOU NEED TO KNOW

• *Prevent delays with good documentation.* One of the reasons that approvals get delayed is the time lost between the original application and the processing of follow-up documents. Any question you respond to with "yes" will need to be verified. You can help speed up the process by including as much supporting documentation as possible with your original application. Does your grandchild receive Social Security? Include a photocopy of the check. Do you have guardianship or court placement? Include court documents—and, of course, a birth certificate or any other paperwork that confirms the child's relationship to you.

• *Make sure you ask about additional medical benefits for children.* Medicaid offers additional benefits to address preventive health care for children. Many people think that because their kids or grandkids are in a Medicaid managed care plan, they shouldn't ask about additional services. But managed care is a delivery system. It doesn't change the benefit to which a child is entitled. (See "Early Periodic Screening, Diagnosis, and Treatment [EPSDT]," below.)

• *Not all doctors accept Medicaid.* Once your grandchild's benefits begin, you will need to find doctors who accept payment through Medicaid. Because of lower reimbursement rates and the paperwork involved, many doctors are reluctant to accept it. If you run into problems, remember that most county hospitals, county clinics, and free clinics are good resources.

EARLY PERIODIC SCREENING, DIAGNOSIS, AND TREATMENT (EPSDT)

What It Is

EPSDT is a benefit of the federal Medicaid program that specifically addresses the needs of children. It is designed to provide financially needy children with preventive health care by detecting and treating early signs of disease or disability and by connecting them with ongoing, comprehensive medical assistance. Federal policy defines the parameters of EPSDT programs, but they are administered by individual state programs whose names and regulations may vary. In California, for instance, EPSDT is handled through a program called Child Health and Disability Prevention (CHDP). Some states give it more user-friendly names like Health Check or Care for Kids. It may have another name in your state. Whatever it's called, EPSDT is a critical benefit for your grandchildren because it provides many services that may not be available to adult Medicaid recipients.

Who Is Eligible

Every child under 21 who is eligible for Medicaid is eligible for federally funded EPSDT benefits, whether they are called that or not. (See "Medicaid," above.) Some states also provide early screening and prevention services to low-income children who are not eligible for Medicaid. If your grandchildren are not eligible for Medicaid, ask state resources if there is a state-funded program that applies to them.

What You Get

Services include free childhood screening and free medically necessary follow-up diagnosis and treatment for conditions found during the EPSDT screens.

Screening

Regular well-baby and well-child checkups are the foundation of EPSDT benefits. These typically include a full unclothed physical exam; assessment of physical and mental health development; vision, hearing, and dental screening; health education; a nutrition check; age-appropriate vaccinations and booster shots; and appropriate or necessary lab tests, including tests for lead poisoning. However, states vary in how well they carry out these requirements.

Diagnosis and Treatment

Your grandchild is entitled to a broad range of free diagnosis and treatment services through EPSDT. Your state should provide "medically necessary" corrective treatment for any physical or mental illness or condition that is suspected or detected during an EPSDT screen, as long as it is covered by federal Medicaid. This means that your state may be required to provide certain services to children even though it may not provide those same services to adult Medicaid recipients. These services can include assessment for and provision of glasses, hearing aids, and medical equipment; dental care to relieve pain and infection; dental health maintenance and teeth restoration; rehabilitation; respiratory care; home health services; and inpatient or outpatient services to evaluate physical or mental illness.

Although each state may have its own definition for "medically necessary," federal law requires every state to provide diagnostic and treatment services "to correct or ameliorate defects and physical and mental illnesses and conditions discovered by the screening services."[14]

Additional Help and Information

State agencies are obligated to inform the caregivers of all eligible children about EPSDT benefits and to make those services available to them. To this end, you should be provided with a list of appropriate providers near you, as well as their addresses. You should also be offered scheduling and transportation assistance, if you need it, for your grandchildren's regularly scheduled checkups.

The Application Process

How It Should Work

Early periodic screening, diagnosis, and treatment is a benefit of the Medicaid program. You shouldn't need to apply for it. You should be offered information on EPSDT services when you apply for Medicaid for your grandchildren. If your grandchild is eligible (and most GAP grandchildren should be), you can schedule an appointment through whichever state or county program administers these services.

Your grandchild's periodic checkups should be scheduled on a regular basis determined by your state. However, you are entitled to request additional screens whenever these are needed to determine the existence of a new disease or condition or whenever an existing condition seems to change or worsen. For instance, if your granddaughter starts to squint in school, you may request a vision screening even if her next scheduled appointment is several months away.

How It Often Works

Grandparents are not always informed about EPSDT benefits, and while federal guidelines require states to use broader standards when providing services to children, some states still apply the stricter adult Medicaid standards and may not offer certain services, even though they are covered by EPSDT.

■ WHAT YOU NEED TO KNOW

• *EPSDT is an important resource for your grandchildren.* Whereas Medicaid is designed to treat illness, EPSDT is designed for early detection and prevention. Without early intervention, many conditions, including mental health problems and learning disabilities, can become more difficult and costly to treat. Make sure to ask about it when you apply for Medicaid.

• *Don't let names confuse you.* Not all eligibility workers recognize the acronym EPSDT—your state program may have another name for it—so ask about *preventive medical benefits* for children: well child care, early screening, treatment, and medically necessary services.

• *Many providers are poorly informed.* There are a number of private Medicaid providers and personnel in county facilities who are not aware of the full extent of early screening and treatment benefits. They may not be aware that additional (interperiodic) screens and checkups are allowed, or they may be reluctant to provide them because reimbursement is slow. They may also mistakenly bill you for services that should be paid for by the state. If this happens, photocopy the bill and send it back to the doctor with a letter of explanation. Always keep a copy for yourself.

• *Many states don't fully implement federal EPSDT regulations.* As with many government programs, there can be a discrepancy between federal EPSDT ideals and state practice. For instance, while mental health assessment and dental care follow-ups are both required by federal law, some state programs may not offer them. If you have problems receiving EPSDT services for your grandchild, you can ask for a hearing. Contact your local Legal Aid or Protection and Advocacy chapters for help (see Appendix A).

• *Ask about state programs.* Some states also provide early screening and prevention services to low-income and medically fragile children who are not eligible for Medicaid. If your grandchildren are not eligible for Medicaid, ask if there is a state-funded program that applies to them.

SUPPLEMENTAL NUTRITIONAL ASSISTANCE PROGRAM (SNAP)

What It Is

The government provides nutritional assistance to needy families through EBT (Electronic Benefit Transfer) cards, electronic debit cards that can be used like money in the grocery store or with other approved vendors. These funds, long known as "food stamps," can be used to buy food or seeds to grow food. You cannot use them to purchase items like diapers, toilet paper, tobacco, alcohol, or pet food.

Who Is Eligible

Many families who receive welfare assistance are also eligible for nutritional assistance. However, your grandchild's eligibility for SNAP, unlike welfare assistance, will be affected by your income and the income of everyone in your household, as well as immigrant status. For purposes of eligibility, a household is a family or group of individuals who live in the same place and buy and prepare food together. If you and your grandchild are *both* receiving welfare assistance, it is possible that you are both entitled to nutritional assistance. However, if your grandchild is getting foster care benefits, you may exclude him from being counted in your household. If he receives basic welfare, both your income and his will be counted on the application.

What You Get

The amount of food stamps you can receive depends on a number of factors, including your income, your resources, how many people are in your household, and the cost of your living expenses, such as rent and utilities. Your eligibility worker should be able to tell you which resources can be counted against your eligibility.

The Application Process

How It Should Work

You can apply for food stamps through your local SNAP office or at your state or local welfare office at the same time you apply for welfare assistance. In some states the application form for food stamps comes as part of the same application package. Many states also allow you to apply online.

■ WHAT YOU NEED TO KNOW

- *Don't let names confuse you.* For years, this program was referred to as Food Stamps. In 2008, the federal program was renamed SNAP (Supplemental Nutrition Assistance Program), and it may go by yet a different name in your state. In California, for instance, it's Cal-Fresh. Whatever it's called in your area, the focus remains the same: nutritional assistance. And it's worth looking into.
- *It always pays to apply.* Many grandparents either are too embarrassed to apply for "food stamps" or believe they won't qualify. If there is any possibility that you and your grandchildren may be eligible for nutritional assistance, apply for it. Raising children is an expensive proposition; you deserve any help you can get.
- *You have a right to a "fair hearing."* Request one if you do not qual-

ify for SNAP and feel you were unfairly denied, if you need to address mistakes or unfair treatment, or if you believe your benefits are too low.

• *Keeping records is necessary.* If you do qualify, keep receipts and bills for all your purchases. You will have to report changes in your income and expenses on a regular basis, and you may need receipts to verify your records.

SPECIAL SUPPLEMENTAL NUTRITION PROGRAM FOR WOMEN, INFANTS, AND CHILDREN (WIC)

What It Is

WIC is a nutrition education and supplemental nutrition program for low-income pregnant women, mothers, infants, and children who have health risks. WIC originates in the U.S. Department of Agriculture and is adminis-tered by either a health or human services agency in each state.

Who Is Eligible

Low-income pregnant women, mothers, infants, and children whose health is at risk are eligible for WIC. Eligibility can continue up to the age of five, provided the child continues to have a health risk and meets the income criteria, and the state has sufficient funding to serve all applicants. Although grandparents are not eligible for these benefits, grandchildren may qualify. Eligibility is determined by your income and the health needs of the child (a drug-exposed infant, for instance, definitely has a health risk).

What You Get

WIC is similar to SNAP in that you get checks, vouchers, or, in some states, EBT cards to be used at the grocery store like money. However, WIC vouch-ers are earmarked for specific foods that support the nutritional needs of the child. For instance, one voucher may be for a dozen eggs, another for a gallon of milk or for infant formula. Those who are eligible also receive educational information about nutrition and child development through a class or a counselor. Finally, you can use WIC as a referral center for other appropriate health care services for your grandchild.

The Application Process

How It Should Work

You can obtain information on how to apply for WIC by calling your county health department or your state social services or welfare office. If they don't handle the WIC program in your area, they can refer you to the agency that does. Once you call, a WIC worker may be able to do a preliminary screening by phone, asking you questions about your income. If you meet these first requirements, the worker will schedule an interview for you and your grandchild.

Three things happen in the interview at the clinic or office. First, you are given a second, more in-depth, screening for income. If you meet this requirement, your grandchild will be screened for "health risk" criteria: An assessment of her diet is made on the basis of what the child ate in the last 24 hours, she is tested for anemia by means of a finger-stick blood test and is weighed and measured, and a health questionnaire on the child is filled out. This package determines whether the child is eligible.

WIC determines eligibility on the spot; you won't have to wait days to find out. In most states you get your first vouchers before you leave the office. However, as with all benefits, delivery varies from state to state. Once you qualify for WIC, you are certified for six months. You will then be recertified every six months until the child is no longer eligible.

How It Often Works

Applying for WIC vouchers involves another appointment, another meeting, another place to haul your grandchild, and more forms to fill out. None of this is made easy for you. Moreover, because WIC is not fully funded, not every child who is technically eligible gets covered. When states cut back, they do so by age, dropping the upper age limit from five years to four or three or even younger.

■ WHAT YOU NEED TO KNOW

If you have a child under the age of five, apply for this! Many grandparents hear about the income qualification and assume they won't qualify. Since WIC often allows income levels higher than welfare, Medicaid, or SNAP, you may still meet the WIC criteria even if you have a retirement income. Even if your grandchild doesn't qualify for this program, WIC can be a good first line of referral to other health care services.

WHERE TO LOOK FOR ADDITIONAL SERVICES IN YOUR STATE

This chapter has reviewed only basic federal assistance that may be available to your grandchildren. You might also look into government-funded Head Start programs as a source of day care as well as early childhood education and socialization for very young grandchildren. Many states and communities have independent programs and organizations that support children and families in need. Survivors of crime victims can often receive financial assistance for funerals or counseling through programs developed to assist this population. State or local public health offices and community health centers may provide free or low-cost health care for children. Religious and charitable organizations like Catholic Charities, Jewish Family Services, and Family Service America may offer help with food, clothing, and transportation. Churches, synagogues, and community centers may sponsor child care and after-school activities, as well as camp scholarships for fixed-income children.

Ask your grandchild's teacher or doctor about additional local resources. Find out if your area has an information and referral line. And don't forget grandparent support groups. In addition to providing emotional support, some grandparent groups help with general assistance, and they are a wonderful source of information.

13

Special Education and Early Intervention

If you've told a child a thousand times and he still does not understand, then it is not the child who is a slow learner.
—*Walter Barbee*[1]

Ever since 1954, when the U.S. Supreme Court ruled to desegregate schools in *Brown v. Board of Education,* American children have enjoyed the right to equal education.[2] But if your grandchild cannot see the blackboard, read the alphabet, remember instructions, or stay in her seat, she cannot take advantage of the education she is entitled to, no matter how good that education may be.

Fortunately, the civil rights movement of the 1960s also drew attention to the rights of the handicapped, including the need of disabled children for equal access to their equal education. Congress therefore passed laws that gave states a financial incentive to offer special resources to kids with disabilities.[3]

Children having serious difficulties in school are entitled to a number of special education programs and services to help them make the most of their public education. Two particular federal laws, or parts of them, apply to children with special education needs:

Section 504 of the Rehabilitation Act of 1973 is a civil rights law. It prohibits discrimination against the disabled in any program that receives federal funds, including schools.[4] If your grandchild has a disability that limits certain activities but does not affect his academic performance, he may be entitled to modifications in the classroom and curriculum through Section 504.

IDEA 2004 (Individuals with Disabilities Education Improvement Act of 2004) requires all states and territories to ensure that all children with disabilities have access to a "free appropriate public education" (FAPE) that emphasizes special education and services "designed to meet their unique needs and prepare them for further education, employment, and independent living." It also requires them to protect the rights of children with disabilities and defines the rights of those children and their parents or guardians or court-appointed educational rights holders.[5] "Appropriate" means that the curriculum meets the special education needs of each child's disability. If your grandchild's disabilities seriously hinder his academic achievement, he may be eligible for special education services through IDEA.

A "free appropriate public education" is a right and an entitlement, not a privilege. It is implemented through a procedure called an IEP, or individualized education program. This is a detailed plan of special services, tailored to the needs of each child, which the school must provide to ensure that the child's education is indeed "appropriate."

The IEP is considered the centerpiece of special education law, and each stage of the special education process is a stepping-stone toward completing it: the assessment of the child through a battery of tests, observations, and reports; meetings of teachers, professionals, and parents (or, in this case, grandparents) to evaluate whether the child qualifies for services and which services would help him; and the IEP itself, which must be carried out by the school or school district.

This process helps determine whether the problems a child is exhibiting are due to a physical, emotional, or learning disability and suggests how an environment might be created that would enable him to benefit from his public school education. This can mean individual tutoring, putting the child in a special class in the current school, or transferring to another school, whether public or private, that can better handle the disability.

"Free appropriate public education. Those are the buzz words," warns one special education commissioner. "You get a compact VW, not a Rolls Royce or a Mercedes."[6] In other words, you get the services that will give your grandchild an even playing field, but not more than that. But an even playing field can mean the difference between getting an education and slipping through the cracks for a child with ADHD or a learning disability. The more you can learn about the special education process and the IEP, the better you can use it as a tool to provide your grandchild with an education that will allow him to learn.

THE SPECIAL EDUCATION PROCESS

The Request

The special education process begins with a written request to your local school. Even if your grandchild is not yet enrolled there, if he is three to five years old, you can contact the principal or someone in charge of special education. If you have any problems, call your state's department of education and ask who in your area is responsible for special education programs for preschoolers with disabilities.

Anyone—a teacher, a therapist, a pediatrician, a parent or guardian, or, in your case, a grandparent—can request a special education evaluation for a child. No matter how small your town is, the school should know about the IEP. Your grandchild may have to go to another school or district for the evaluation—some areas have created a consortium among several schools to handle this—but you must still start the process with a written request to your local school. Date the letter and keep a copy for your files. This request will start a clock ticking; the school district is required to process eligibility for special education within a prescribed time frame. That time frame is dictated by state law, and many school districts fall behind their prescribed schedules. (The schedule in this chapter represents California law. Your own state's time frame may be different, so find out what it is. Don't let the school drag the process out so that your grandchild falls further behind.)

The Evaluation or Assessment Plan

Once the school receives your request, it has 15 days (in California) to send you a plan for how it will evaluate your grandchild. This is a key step; don't take it lightly. The kind of testing done in the assessment will determine the kinds of services your grandchild is eligible to receive. If the child needs psychological counseling or speech therapy but those tests are not included in the assessment plan, they won't be considered in the IEP.

What testing do you want the school to do? If you don't know, take the plan to someone who can help you. You need to make sure the school is offering the right assessment for this child at this age and with these particular needs. Assessments are expensive; with budgets tight, school districts do try to cut corners where they can. You have to be the child's best advocate. Persistence and perseverance do pay off. If the assessment plan is adequate, sign and return it. If not, write in the additional tests you want before you send it back.

The Actual Assessment or Evaluation

Once you return the signed plan, the school district has 60 calendar days (in California) to complete the assessment, which is a multidisciplinary evaluation usually conducted by a school psychologist, teacher, educational diagnostician, social worker, and other evaluators. This evaluation includes medical, educational, psychological, and sociological components. Try to get as much input into this process as possible. If you think the school's assessment is inadequate, and if you can afford it, you can have your own assessment done privately.

The Eligibility Meeting

Once the assessment is complete, the school district will schedule a meeting to determine if the child is eligible for special education services. However, some state and local agencies combine the eligibility meeting and the IEP meeting (see below) into a single conference.

What Determines Eligibility?

According to federal regulations, all "children with disabilities" are eligible for special education and related services. This includes children who have been evaluated as being mentally retarded, physically handicapped, health impaired, or emotionally disturbed, or as having specific learning disabilities. However, terms like "emotionally disturbed" and "learning disabled" are hard to define, and the final criteria for special education eligibility vary from state to state.

You might think your grandchild is learning disabled—and by many standards she may be—but the child must fit your state's criteria to be eligible for services. For instance, if your state defines a learning-disabled child as one of normal intelligence who is two years behind her age group, but your dyslexic granddaughter is only one year behind, she may not qualify for special education in that state.

Even if your grandchild is not eligible for an IEP through the Individuals with Disabilities Education Improvement Act, she should be able to get certain classroom modifications through Section 504. These might include having your grandchild placed at the front of the classroom, allowing her to use a tape recorder in class, or giving her more time to complete certain tests and assignments.

If it is determined that your grandchild does have a disability that makes her eligible for an IEP, the school district or public agency has up to 60 days (in California) from the date you return the signed assessment plan in which to complete assessments, hold an IEP meeting to determine eligibility, and put an appropriate program into place.

The IEP Meeting

The IEP meeting itself can take place in any number of places—a district office, a hospital, your home—but it is most commonly held in your grandchild's own school. It should be held at a time and place that are mutually agreeable to school personnel and to you, as the child's guardian.

The IEP is based on a team concept: A group of professionals work with the parents (or grandparents) and, if appropriate, the child, to determine what services his special education will include. The team players are the school administrator or principal, the child's teacher, the school nurse, and a psychologist. Federal law also requires that a general education and special education teacher be present at all IEP meetings.[7]

During the IEP meeting this team will examine your grandchild's test results, profiles, class work, teacher reports, nurse's reports, and any other material that is presented as pertinent. If a psychologist or a doctor needs to present information in person, this is where it happens. If a medical doctor is scheduled to be present, try to have your grandchild's own doctor there as well. Remember, you are an important part of this team. As primary caregiver, you are the one who knows your grandchild best, and no services can be provided without your consent. You are allowed to present any information or reports and bring any persons to an IEP who have relevant information to provide regarding your grandchild's educational performance. This can include people who assist your grandchild with homework, a psychologist or educational diagnostician, a therapist, or other mental health providers.

Several things are decided at the IEP meeting: goals and objectives, placement, related services, and, for some children, transition services. The IEP form will be filled out on the basis of these decisions, and the IEP will become the blueprint or game plan for your grandchild's education. At many meetings, the school district has a proposed IEP already written. By asking for a copy of it in advance, you can follow along better at the meeting, raise any questions or concerns you might have, and make suggestions to improve the plan.

Goals and Objectives

If your grandchild is found eligible for special education services, the next thing to decide is what kind of program and services are needed. What are your grandchild's specific disabilities? What does he need to learn to catch up to other children his age? These are the questions that must be addressed at the IEP meeting. These questions should be answered with specific goals and objectives and a schedule for measuring whether or not they are being achieved. For instance, if Carrie is a bright fifth grader who tests at a second-grade reading level, she clearly needs help with reading. But her IEP should say more than "Carrie will get help with reading." Instead, Carrie's IEP goals might state that "Carrie will be able to read at a third-grade level by the end of the first semester. By the end of the year, Carrie will be reading on a fourth-grade level." The goals should also state which test will measure this progress.

Goals and objectives are critical in deciding which kind of placement and services your grandchild is eligible for in the coming year. Make sure they can be measured objectively. A teacher's observation or opinion is not an objective measurement. Also, make sure that your grandchild has a clear IEP goal/objective in each area of need.

Placement

The law requires that each child be placed in the "least restrictive environment." That means having the child in as regular a school program as possible while accommodating his special needs. Special options can range from extra help in a mainstream class to residential placement. Other possibilities include special day classes, a resource specialist for tutoring, a state school, or, occasionally, a private school paid for by the school district. If your grandchild does need a special school and there are none in your area, he may be sent out of the district.

Related Services

If a child qualifies for special education, school districts are also supposed to provide certain additional services to help her come up to speed. "Related services" can include speech and language services, psychological counseling, special readers, tutoring, medical services in school, parent training, physical and occupational therapy, adaptive physical education, and even transportation if you live far from a special education program.

Transition Services

The IEP is designed not only to help disabled children graduate but to help older children with disabilities make the transition to life after school. Thus, an IEP could include not only special instruction but employment, vocational, or college counseling, certain community experiences, and even instruction in specific daily living skills like filling out applications, handling money, and finding living arrangements. Starting at no later than

16 years old (and sometimes at 14 or younger) your grandchild's IEP should include a plan for the transition services he will need to move on in life.

Remember, although the IEP works on a team concept, it is also a negotiation session. Your concern is your grandchild's needs, but the school must focus on hundreds of children and must do so with dwindling funds. Since it is expensive to put kids in special classes and nonpublic schools, a school district does resist. After all, the less they give you, the more remains in their budget. On the other hand, the more prepared you are, the more you can get out of the system.

The IEP

The product of the IEP process is the actual IEP, the written individualized education program that you as the child's guardian must approve and sign before services can take effect. Read the IEP carefully before you sign it. Make sure it does what it is meant to do. Ask yourself the following questions:

Is it comprehensive? A good IEP should cover every area of your grandchild's development, including behavior, socialization, communication, self-help, academic, and motor skills.

Is it specific? Are goals and objectives clearly stated in terms of objective, observable, and measurable behavior?

Is it sequential? Does it offer a solid step-by-step plan to teach your grandchild what she needs to learn?

Is it realistic and appropriate? Does it match your grandchild's current abilities? Does it encourage growth at a reasonable rate?

Is it understandable? Is it written in language that you can comfortably follow and discuss?

Was it mutually developed? In other words, were you an active part of the IEP team and does the final plan reflect your concerns?

Is it designed to close the gap between the child's ability and her achievement?

Remember, the IEP is key to your grandchild's education; you want to make sure the door it opens is the right one.

Don't Do This Yourself

Even the most sophisticated, resourceful grandparent can find the IEP process overwhelming. You have to tell strangers how badly off your grandchild is, and that can be hard to do without getting emotionally involved. The forms can be confusing, and the process can drag on until you run out of patience. It is good to learn the terminology and the process, but you have enough to do already without having to learn all the detailed procedures of educational law and the difference between various types of assessment plans.

The individual who helps you negotiate an IEP with your grandchild's school could be an attorney or advocate, a therapist or social worker, even another grandparent or a friend. A local education attorney or advocate knows the ropes: whom to ask, what to ask, and what to ask for. She may have even worked with this IEP team before. An educational therapist, a psychologist, or a social worker can evaluate the assessment plan and help fill out the IEP form with your wish list. These professionals have a better grasp of what are reasonable goals for your grandchild at his age and with his particular psychological and educational background. If you can't find or afford an advocate, look for another grandparent or parent who has been through this before; ask that parent to go to the IEP meeting with you. At the very least, take a friend or relative for support. Despite what anyone may tell you, you do have the right to have someone there.

Preparing for the IEP Meeting

The more information you have before your first IEP, the fewer problems you are likely to encounter. Here are some things you can do to prepare yourself for the IEP meeting:

- *Learn about your and your grandchild's rights.* Your grandchild has rights and so do you, as the primary caregiver or guardian. Get copies of federal rules and regulations (IDEA 2004 and Section 504), your state rules and regulations for special education, and the policies in effect in your school district. Remember, the only interpretation that ultimately counts is the federal one.

- *Find out the chain of command in your school district.* If you are not satisfied with the outcome of the IEP meeting and need to go higher up, you will already know whom to go to.
- *Keep records.* Write down the names and numbers of everyone you talk to. They could be helpful later on.
- *Review your grandchild's school records.* Go to the school and photocopy everything that is in the child's cumulative and confidential reports. You may have to check in different departments to get all of them. If the child has ever been in any kind of facility, get their records as well. Copy everything: handwritten notes, notes scribbled on the folder or jacket, any work the child has done. You are arming yourself on all fronts. You can also request that the school district provide you with copies of all its records. Make your request in writing, and the school district has to provide you all its records from all sources within a reasonable period of time (no more than 45 days after receiving the request).[8] The district cannot charge you copying costs if you are below the poverty line or on welfare, or if the cost would prevent you from having the records
- *Speak with the psychologist.* Find out who the psychologist is and get her reports on your grandchild. Be nice about this; presume that the psychologist is doing the best job she can for the child. If you are using an advocate, he will know how to ask the right questions.
- *Request your own copy of the assessment report.* You can also prepare yourself for your grandchild's IEP meeting by asking to receive a copy of the assessment report prior to the IEP. This way, you can read the report and note any questions you may want to have answered at the meeting.
- *If you have had an outside assessment done, plan to bring it.* Or, if possible, bring along the expert who did the assessment; he or she may be able to provide additional information. Make sure you notify the school in advance that you will be presenting your own report.
- *Gather outside information.* Collect medical records and any school or test records the school district may not have. Because reports don't tell you everything about a child, be sure to bring in real-life examples of your grandchild's abilities and disabilities in different areas. Talk to other adults who come into contact with your grandchild—doctors, social workers, clergy members, even family and neighbors. Ask them to

put their comments and observations in writing. Submit this information for the assessment.

• *Set your own goals for your grandchild.* If you let the school district define all of your grandchild's goals and objectives, it may only offer minimal services and will probably not address all your grandchild's needs. Make a list of what things your grandchild can do and what you think he should learn during the school year. Get blank copies of the IEP forms, photocopy them, and fill them in. Focus on your goals for your grandchild and how you want them to be accomplished. Does he have problems hopping or jumping? Ask for adaptive physical education. This is your wish list.

• *Think about placement.* What do you want for your grandchild? Talk to someone who knows your school district and ask the following questions: What special classrooms are available? What do they offer? Where are there special schools? Visit any classroom or school where you think they might place your grandchild. Interview the teacher. If you're not happy with the placement, take in your own plan. You may have a fight on your hands, but it could be worth it. You might even be able to get your grandchild placed in a private school, but that is a difficult proposition.

• *Ask for therapy.* One important goal that is often overlooked is psychological counseling. Being in a special education classroom, as helpful as it is, carries a stigma that is hard on children. Their self-esteem is low. Other children may tease them. Always try to get mental health testing and psychological counseling into your grandchild's IEP, and make sure that it is with a trained therapist. The school may view sessions with a guidance counselor as therapy, but many guidance counselors may not be qualified to deal with the issues your grandchild could be experiencing.

• *Consider nonacademic activities.* Lunch, recess, physical education, and activities like art and music are important parts of the school day. Make sure your grandchild's IEP lets her take advantage of the nonacademic part of school as well.

• *Carefully consider having your grandchild at the meeting.* Despite what anyone may tell you, you are entitled to have the child present. The question is, Do you want to? The IEP process can be devastating. Personally, I don't recommend that a young child be present at an IEP meeting. Perhaps a high school student may be confident enough to provide some input, but I can't think of a good reason to have an elementary school child present. These children have such fragile self-esteem that they can't help but be affected by everyone talking about their problems. However, your grandchild must eventually learn to become his own advocate.

● *Be vigilant.* In so many arenas you have had to step gingerly with bureaucracy; this is one place you must be willing to push. Just because public schools have a duty to identify children who need special education doesn't mean they always do so. Children get lost in the school system. The ones who are quiet and nice may get C's or D's and yet be passed along without services.

Don't back down. Remember, it's the squeaky wheel that gets the grease, and the people who go down to the school and insist on the services they need that get them. So, even if you have an advocate, be vigilant.

During the IEP Meeting

● *Be confident.* Your image may affect how school personnel respond to you. Bring your own set of rules, regulations, and supporting material. Have your grandchild's file organized neatly and in chronological order; keep state and federal regulations in a separate folder. This way you also look prepared. Speak clearly and maintain eye contact. And remember, this committee is paid to work for you and your grandchild; they are not dispensing favors. Special education is a right, not a privilege.

● *Have people sign in.* Pass around a sign-in sheet at the beginning of the meeting. This will let you address everyone by name.

● *Ask questions.* Especially when you don't understand something, ask about it. You have a right to simple explanations of anything that is unclear to you.

● *Repeat what you are asking for.* Do this as often as necessary. Remember, you're not there to discuss the dwindling school budget. You're there to make sure your child gets an appropriate education.

• *If necessary, request another meeting.* If you cannot come to an agreement, are running out of time, or need more time to think, you have the right to request another meeting. You do not have to make a decision at that moment.

• *Don't sign an IEP until you understand and agree with it.* Remember that you do not have to sign an unsatisfactory IEP. If you do not agree with the school's evaluation, you can get an independent evaluation and request a new meeting based on it. You can also file an appeal through a mediation process or a "due process hearing" (see below). If you have an IEP you like, and the school wants to change it by reducing services or taking away transportation, for instance, don't sign it, and your current IEP will remain in force.

"You are in a powerful position," says Jill Rowland, director of special education programs for the Alliance for Children's Rights.[9] "If you don't like a change, don't sign the document. The onus is on the school district to convince parents to change or to file a due process to defend the program as being appropriate. It's one of the only places parents have some power, but if they don't know about it, they can't exercise it."

After the IEP Meeting

• *Request your own copy of the final IEP.*

• *Follow your grandchild's progress closely.* Periodically ask the teachers for a progress report. Remember, you can initiate changes or a review if your grandchild is not improving. You can also request another IEP meeting.

• *Ask teachers what you can do at home to help.* Many skills your grandchild will be learning at school can be practiced at home.

• *Keep records.* Record anything you want to ask about or discuss with the school, all meetings and phone conversations you want to remember, and any information that may be useful in future reviews and evaluations. It is easy to forget what you don't write down.

• *Try to resolve any problems you have with the school within the school district.* On the other hand, if you cannot come to an agreement with school officials and your grandchild is not being properly supported, you can file an appeal.

The Appeal Process

If the final IEP is not acceptable to you and you cannot resolve the issue with the school district, you can appeal. Some states offer a mediation process first, but any issues that cannot be resolved in mediation will be taken to a due process hearing. Likewise, if the IEP is not being followed, you can file a formal complaint with your state board of education, the U.S. Department of Education, or the Office of Civil Rights and start an investigation. You are entitled to be present when your complaint comes before the board of education. Sometimes, if the school district thinks you will fight them all the way to a hearing, they may give you what you want—it's cheaper. If the due process hearing is not satisfactory, the appeal process can go on to a U.S. district court and, in some cases, up to the U.S. Supreme Court.

If you do start the appeal process, you may want to consult an attorney or advocate. Most states have Protection and Advocacy agencies, although they may go by different names. You can find a complete listing online (see Appendix A, Parenting and Education Resources, National Disability Rights Network). So look around before you decide you can't afford representation. And don't be afraid to "rock the boat." A free *appropriate* public education is a right that belongs to your grandchild; you have a right to make sure that what is provided is appropriate.

The Review Process

At least once a year, the school must schedule an annual meeting to review and revise your grandchild's IEP. The IEP may also be revised anytime you see a need for revision and make a request in writing. States may have their own timelines for reviewing and revising the IEP and for reassessing a child to see if her needs are being met and progress is being made, and to determine what changes are needed as she gets older. This is not a bad thing. Frequent academic testing can help you closely monitor your grandchild's progress. If she is not making adequate progress, this information can help you argue for more services. You can also request, in writing, that your grandchild be tested more often than the scheduled timeline. In the letter, describe your concerns and the reasons you are requesting the meeting.

EARLY INTERVENTION AND SPECIAL EDUCATION SERVICES FOR INFANTS AND TODDLERS WITH DISABILITIES

One of the wonderful things about IDEA is the possibility of early intervention, that is, of addressing the needs of disabled children before they enter the school system and start to fall behind. Federal law extends special education assistance to children beginning at birth if they have an established risk condition such as Down syndrome, or a developmental delay. Children who are at risk for developing disabilities, such as drug-exposed infants or babies born prematurely, are also eligible in a number of places, although this varies state by state.

The goal of early intervention is to identify and treat problems and delays in children as soon as possible. This can be as simple as prescribing glasses for a three-year-old or as intensive as complete physical therapy for an infant with cerebral palsy. The theory is that the more special assistance a child receives early on, when the rate of learning is fastest, the fewer the special education services he may need later in life.

The process of applying for early intervention is similar to applying for the IEP and involves the following stages:

The Request

If your grandchild is under three, different states task different agencies to provide these services. In California, these services are provided by local regional centers. Anyone can request an early start assessment from their local regional center; this should be done in writing. If your child is in foster care, you should ask your social worker to also do a referral at the same time you are doing your own.

The Assessment

Your grandchild will be evaluated by a team of professionals, which may include a psychologist and an occupational or a physical therapist as well as other experts, depending on the rules and regulations of your state. You are an important part of this team and should participate as much as you can in this process. Many of the preparation suggestions for the IEP apply here (see above).

The Plan

If your grandchild is eligible for early intervention services, the assessment team will create an IFSP (individualized family service plan). Like the IEP, this plan describes the child's developmental level, the goals to be achieved, which services the child will receive, where and when she will receive these services, and what steps will be taken to ease the child's transition into school or another program.

Unlike the IEP, which focuses on the individual student, the IFSP addresses the whole family. The philosophy is that the best way to meet the needs of a small child is to work with the family. This can include family counseling, respite care, and educational services to help everyone understand and cope with your grandchild's disability.

The Services

Early intervention services may be offered through public or private agencies in a variety of settings: clinics, hospitals, neighborhood day care centers, the local health department, even your home. All early intervention services provided under the IDEA are supposed to be free of cost. Again, each state develops its own policies for carrying out the IDEA. You will need to find out about the specific policies in your state. The National Information Center for Children and Youth with Disabilities (NICHCY) publishes free resource sheets listing agencies and contact people in each state (see "Parenting and Education Resources" in Appendix A for more information).

AND IT'S ANOTHER NOTEBOOK!

Lots of paperwork is generated with special needs children: assessment reports, IFSPs, IEPs, medical forms, phone numbers, conferences, growth milestones, immunizations, therapy reports, and so on. The more organized you are, the better you can protect your grandchild's right to a free and equal education.

What to Keep in Your Child's Home File

- A copy of IDEA 2004 and its regulations.
- A copy of your state's rules and regulations on special education.
- A copy of the school's IEP procedures.
- A "chain of command" list. Keep a list or chart of the chain of command within the school system, beginning at the local level and ending with state and federal agencies. Include addresses and telephone numbers for easy reference.
- A list of school and IEP players. Every year, list your grandchild's teacher, school, principal, and psychologist, as well as any related services personnel, special education teachers, the school district superintendent, school board members, and the special education administrator.
- Copies of all school records, including the child's cumulative records, psychological reports, and any other papers the school district might have about your grandchild. Keep them chronologically, with the most recent year on top.
- Report cards.
- Copies of test results and recommendations from independent assessments.
- All written (including handwritten) letters and notes to and from school personnel.
- All written communication with outside professionals regarding your grandchild's unique needs.
- Dated notes on parent–teacher conferences.
- Dated notes you have taken during conversations with the child's physician and other professionals who see your grandchild.
- Dated notes on all telephone conversations with school personnel or others regarding your grandchild.
- A list of any medications being given to your grandchild at home and at school as authorized by the child's physician. Include the kind of medicine and dosage information. In addition, note prescription numbers and any changes in dosage or reactions.

ADDITIONAL RESOURCES

There are many kinds of support and information services out there for families with disabled children, from public agencies to support groups for families of children with disabilities. Also, many states have published manuals that explain their special education and related services for children with disabilities. Contact your state department of education or any of the groups or organizations listed in Appendix A for more information.

ONE LAST WORD: AIM HIGH

A disability does not have to be a sentence to failure. It's not that these children can't learn—many are very smart—but they need to learn differently. Give them goals and aim high. The IEP offers transition services for adjusting to life after high school, and Section 504 of the Rehabilitation Act of 1973 prohibits discrimination against disabled applicants or students at schools that receive federal funds. There is financial aid and special programming even at many top colleges and universities. Audio textbooks, extended time for testing, recording devices, computers, and interpreters for students with hearing problems are just a few of the modifications that are helping disabled teenagers participate and succeed on American campuses.

"Go for doctor, lawyer, not secretary," said one special education attorney, who is himself dyslexic. "The [school] will want to put them into bricklaying, truck driving. Don't let it happen."[10]

SECTION III

Strength in Numbers

14

Their Arms about Us

FINDING AND FORMING SUPPORT GROUPS

"GAP is a place where I can go as a grandmother and let my hair down and scream and holler and say what I feel. It is a shoulder to cry on."

"GAP is a place you come to when you reach the end of your rope. Three years in court keeps you from talking about things, and you need to vent. This was the first place we were allowed to sit and cry and tell our story."

"It doesn't matter here whether you're poor or rich, black or white. We become a family here. They have become my family."

"There is no place like this. I lived in constant fear of snapping. I come here and all these mothers start picking me up and, next thing you know, I'm whole again."

"I came in here and I was a beat person. I was a rug. I'm not a rug anymore. I'm a strong person now because of GAP. I'm a human being."

"Instead of aging, I've become younger. I don't look younger, but inside

I feel like a very young person. I can cope with anything now—and
I am."

"Until I found GAP, I was just falling down a vast crevice, hitting my
arms and legs along the way. Then I found them and it was like falling onto the softest, warmest down comforter you could dream of.
When I have those stormy winter nights with the children, I use that
comforter. It belongs to me."

There are many reasons why I urge grandparents to seek out support
groups, as I have repeatedly done throughout this book. Each of these reasons comes back to the same root: While you are sacrificing everything
to help your grandchildren, you need someone to help you. A GAP group
lets you look out for one another.

A group is a fallout shelter, a place for people to come together when
everything seems to be raining down on their heads and exploding
around them. It is the best antidote to the overwhelming feelings of loneliness. It cuts isolation. You can cry and yell in a group and not be judged.
You can make friends who understand you because they have been there.
You can go to a meeting and sit next to another grandfather who is angry
at a son who won't parent or another grandmother who is frustrated with
her granddaughter for disrupting her life. You can unload your concerns
without criticism. It lets you see how normal your feelings are.

A group is a living library. You can find guidance from the experiences other people have had in similar situations. Someone who has
already raised a grandchild to age 15 can give you specific feedback on
your five-year-old. This is also a source for practical information, like
phone numbers of attorneys and helpful social workers, and for assistance in navigating issues like obtaining custody or government assistance for the kids.

A group can also be a kind of way station, a place where basic needs
can be gratified through, for example, a clothing exchange, a ride to a
doctor's appointment, a new friend who might watch the kids for an hour.
One support group in Las Vegas organized themselves to pay for medical
exams and eyeglasses for disadvantaged grandparents. "We're not doing
for the child," said its executive director. "We are doing for the grandparents so they can do for the child.[1]

FINDING A GROUP IN YOUR AREA

There are hundreds of grandparent groups running in the United States, and new ones are constantly cropping up. Some of them are chapters or offshoots of larger organizations; others are local, organized by individual grandparents, social workers, therapists, nurses, churches, and even teachers. A number of support groups offer additional services, including the dispensing of newsletters, resource directories, and how-to manuals; hotlines; and emergency assistance with basic needs like food, housing, and financial assistance. And many are active in political and legislative advocacy.

One of the easiest ways to find a local support group is to search online for "grandparents as parents" or "grandparents raising grandchildren" and "meeting." Your search may result in event listings, newspaper articles, or the websites of the groups themselves. If you are not computer savvy, or don't find anything online, check some of the resources in Appendix A; some may be able to point you to a group in your area. You should also call your local child guidance clinic or family service agency to see if the staff knows of any grandparent groups that are just starting up. If not, you may be able to convince them of the need to start one or to help you organize one.

STARTING YOUR OWN GAP GROUP

Before Your First Meeting

There are many kinds of grandparent groups across the country. Some focus on emotional support, some on basic needs and political action, and some on a combination of the three. Some of these groups are run by grandparents, others by social workers and therapists. Each, however, has had to resolve some of the same issues to get up and running.

Identify Your Members

The first step is identifying your target population. Although GAP stands for Grandparents As Parents, our membership extends beyond grandparents who are actually raising their grandchildren. We take grandparents who are fighting for visitation as well as grandparents whose grandchildren were returned to their parents by the system. Aunts, uncles, and cousins come to our meetings, as do older siblings who are raising younger siblings. We've even had a unrelated Big Sister join us—anyone who is raising someone else's child. I don't believe in turning away anyone who can benefit from the information, education, and support GAP offers. On the other hand, we do occasionally narrow our focus by language (we have several Spanish-speaking groups) or grandchild population. We have a few groups devoted to relatives who are raising teenagers and need a very particular kind of support. So who do you want to reach and how do you plan to focus?

Get the Word Out

Once you determine the focus of your GAP group, get the ball rolling by talking it up. Word of mouth does wonders. You never know who might know another grandparent raising a grandchild, and people strike up conversations all the time in the market, the bank, the park, a doctor's office. In fact, most of our grandparents have GAP business cards. If they see a grandparent with a grandchild in a store, at a school meeting, an Al-Anon meeting, or even on the street, they pass them out. One grandmother heard about us through a garage sale. Her mother had bought a whole box of used twin sheets, and the seller asked why she needed so many. "I have a crazy daughter who's raising her grandchildren," she told him. And he told her about GAP.

There are also formal ways to spread the word:

• *Use the Internet.* The quickest way to get the word out is by creating a presence on the Internet. In minutes, you can create a page for your group on Facebook, Google+, or any other social networking sites that are currently popular. Linking to people you know will take word-of-mouth promotion to a new level of digital speed. Likewise, website domains can often be leased for under $10 a year. You can launch your home page with little more than the name of the group, your mission, and the date of your first meeting. This way you will be easy to find if someone searches for grandparent support groups in your area.

You can also post news and links about meetings on a variety of other sites. I see notices for GAP meetings showing up on middle school websites, senior discount sites, event boards, and online radio shows. Think of the Internet as a virtual town center. Where would you hand out flyers for a meeting? Those places have websites, and many post announcements of interest to their readers.

• *Use your community.* You may not know other grandparents in your situation, but there are people who do. Contact local pediatricians, hospitals, social workers, attorneys, schools, churches, and synagogues. Tell them your plans and ask them to give your name and contact information (phone, e-mail, website) to any grandparents they know. They cannot give you a grandparent's name—that's confidential—but they can give out your name or even send out a prepared letter or e-mail. Their offices are also good places to post flyers, if you get permission first.

• *Use the media.* Not only are your local newspaper, radio, and television stations a source of local news, they are your link to other isolated grandparents, especially those who aren't yet computer savvy. There are two ways to get the word out through the media: meeting announcements and articles.

Most newspapers and radio stations have calendar listings of upcoming events. This is a simple way to spread the word. One group sent news releases to as many papers as possible, then followed up with a phone call to confirm. If you do this, be sure to include your name and contact information on your release.

A more challenging, but more effective, approach is the human interest story. Reporters are always on the lookout for personal stories that tie into a social trend. Contact a local newspaper and ask if they would like to do a story on your family. Make sure the article states that you are interested in starting a group for grandparents and includes a contact number. Do the same thing with local radio and television stations.

Encourage Grandfathers to Come

Many grandparent groups seem to be comprised mostly of women. Men are traditionally less inclined to seek out help and support, particularly men of an older generation. They may feel they don't need to talk about their problems or believe they should be able to cope without outside help. But grandfathers do need support, and we have had grandfathers and uncles come to GAP even before their wives did, not to mention single granddads, who are raising grandkids on their own. Like grand-mothers, they benefit from meeting others who have similar feelings and experiences. Some grandfathers even find it helps their marriage to come and learn coping skills as a couple.

When you talk to grandfathers, assure them that they are welcome and that their input is important. And then be patient. A grandmother might come alone every week for months before the grandfather comes; then one meeting might hook him. Your group will benefit from the valu-able perspective that grandfathers offer.

Where Will You Meet?

You will need a location for your meetings. Contact churches, libraries, senior citizens' centers, schools, hospitals, and any other community buildings that have space. If you get a newspaper or radio station inter-ested, mention that you're looking for a donated meeting room. You'll be surprised how many people in the community come through for this type of program.

Word of mouth works, too. Talk it up. Don't be afraid to tell people what you need and to ask for it. One group approached their county coun-cil of churches and found a church where they could use a kitchen and a nursery. Another grandmother attended a parenting class at her grand-child's school and received permission to use a classroom for weekly meetings. The teacher even had her class leave valentines for the grand-parents who use their desks at night.

A word about chairs: Look for a room that already has chairs and/or couches. Also try to find a variety of chairs: Some grandparents are over-weight and need comfortable chairs whereas others have back problems and need sturdy support.

When Will You Meet?

Scheduling is tricky for grandparents, particularly scheduling something for themselves. Many work in the day and may not be able to find or afford a baby-sitter in the evening. Ask grandparents about times when you first contact them, and do the best you can for this first meeting. You won't please everyone, but try for a majority.

Will You Have Child Care?

From the beginning, GAP has offered child care at most evening meetings. Many grandparents cannot afford baby-sitters and have no one to watch their grandchildren. Unless they can solve this problem, they will find it impossible to attend meetings, no matter when you schedule them. You will reach your widest population of grandparents and will be able to help the most people if you make it as easy as possible for them to attend. That means child care.

When you talk to grandparents, ask if they will need child care to attend a group meeting and, if so, how many children they will be bringing. Perhaps you or the other grandparents know someone who would be willing to baby-sit during meetings. Sometimes you can find a volunteer from a church or temple or even a college student from a local child development program who might be able to get class credit for this. You might consider rotating the responsibility among the grandparents who regularly bring grandchildren to the group meeting. (You might consider having name tags for the children so the baby-sitter can call them by name. Make sure sitters know not to release children to anyone but their grandparents.)

Will You Charge for Meetings?

I think it is critical that support groups be free of charge. Otherwise, they just become one more place where grandparents have to give. Group should be a place where they can receive. Many grandparents are on a fixed income. They don't think about their own mental health needs, they think about the needs of their grandchild. If they have extra money one month, they'll buy shoes and a haircut for their grandchildren before doing anything for themselves. Charging for meetings only creates one more barrier to people receiving the help they need. That said, some groups do have a donation box or envelope. Those who can contribute do, and the money goes to planning group events or to helping families in need.

The First Meeting

Here you are. You've found a meeting place and selected the time, the kids are coloring down the hall, and you are looking at a sea of faces in front of you. You have a few more things to consider . . .

Your Nerves

If you're not used to speaking in front of people, you may be nervous at this first meeting. The thoughts may tumble past, one after the other: "How do I start? What do I say? Will all the grandparents get along?" Relax. These are normal thoughts and feelings. Regardless of the group composition—age, race, income, and so on—you are all there for the same reason: You are all dealing with grandchildren in one way or another. That is the focus. This is about emotional and moral support. You are not facing strangers; you are facing future friends.

The Welcome

Introduce yourself. Welcome everyone. Restate the reason for getting together. Stress the importance of confidentiality. Share briefly about yourself: whether or not you are a grandparent, how many children you are raising, why you have them, how long you have had them, your marital status. Let others do the same. Once grandparents start talking, the group takes off.

For many grandparents, this will be their first opportunity to meet others in the same predicament and to express their feelings and talk about issues and concerns. There is a tremendous sense of relief the first time you walk into a room filled with people who will understand and accept you. Some, however, may not choose to talk until they feel more comfortable in the group setting. They may be perfectly happy just listening. Let them know that they are welcome even if they keep silent. And don't worry—each grandparent will wade in at his or her own pace.

Consider using name tags for this first meeting. It helps to connect names and faces in case more than a few people show up. On the other hand, don't be disappointed if you only get one or two the first night. Those two people still need help and will often become part of your core group. Be patient and persistent. Some groups grow slowly, but they do grow.

Group Decisions

During this first meeting you will want to make several decisions:

- *When will you meet?* Will the group keep this scheduled time? How often will it meet? I find that once a week works best, although consistency of meetings is probably more important than frequency. If the group can't meet weekly, schedule a meeting for twice a month or once a month, but make it something reliable to look forward to.

- *How long will meetings be?* Small groups do not necessarily need less time than long groups. Sometimes three grandparents can take up as much time as 12, depending on the number and nature of crises in the room. I find that two to three hours gives everyone a sense of space to share without feeling rushed.

- *Format:* What format will you use? Will you start with all members recapping their week, or will you start with whomever is in crisis or might have to leave early? Let the group decide what format is most comfortable, and recognize that it may change from time to time. One thing I do recommend is setting aside a few minutes for business items and announcements midway through the meeting; this way you catch people who come late and the ones who must leave early.

- *Time-limited or open-ended?* The majority of therapy groups are limited to a set number of weeks and don't allow new members after the first or second session. That was my plan when I started GAP. However, I soon realized that the issues grandparents encounter are much too complex and ongoing to be handled in a limited time frame. All of my groups are open-ended, with new members joining at any time. I have a policy that everyone is welcome, and I never turn anyone away. When new grandparents come into the group, they get great support and guidance from the ones who have been there longer. The grandparents are wonderful about helping each other, and that is one of the joys of the group.

- *Refreshments:* Will you have them? How will you handle them? If you plan to take turns, a sign-up sheet is helpful. If you prefer to pitch into a kitty with one person responsible for buying the refreshments, consider rotating the responsibility every few months.

- *Clean up:* Will you have a volunteer cleanup committee to leave the room in shape? Rotate that, too.

Don't forget to have a sign-in sheet for a directory, exchange names and addresses, and keep a box of tissues handy!

Once You're Under Way

Attendance

Attendance is a changeable thing with grandparents. You will find that a core group will come to each meeting without fail. They will become your educators, helping each other out. They may even become politically active, pursuing changes that might not help their grandchildren but could save someone else's. Other grandparents will come only occasionally. Perhaps they work and can't take time off. Maybe they have medical appointments, sick grandchildren, unreliable transportation, or poor health. Encourage other members to call them to see how they're doing. Let them know they're missed. I've even had grandparents who couldn't come to meetings at all because they had tiny babies or lacked transportation. We've still kept them in the GAP loop, and even connected two home-bound grandmothers as phone buddies. They can't get to group yet, but they're still a part of our community.

Inevitably, a few people may drop out if this is not what they are looking for. Groups are not for everyone.

Participation

It is important that everyone at a meeting has time to share. Some grandparents may not be as verbal as others. Encourage quiet, shy grandparents to participate; as time goes by, they may become more comfortable sharing their feelings. At times, you may have to gently and politely interrupt one grandparent to give others a chance to talk.

A wonderful part of a group is that members benefit from each other's experiences, as well as from the support given and received. It's important to share positive experiences as well as negative experiences, because you learn from both.

Be Patient with Evolution

It is tempting, when you give support and advice, to push for quick changes. It is easy to become impatient with people who seem to be stuck in a situation and yet continue to suffer because of it. But change rarely comes quickly or easily, particularly where the heart is involved. Ultimately, grandparents will make the changes that they can in the time frame they can handle—and no sooner. I have heard grandparents talk for two years before they could take any action, such as getting an adult child out of the house. As a group, you can only support and encourage them. Be there when they need to cry and when they want to laugh. When they're ready to make a change, they will do it. But remember, it will be in their time frame.

There are also situations that have no answers, no clear course of action. Sometimes the only thing to do is talk, cry, and feel the understanding of people who have been there. To air your feelings, to see them as natural, and to know you're not alone and not crazy is the beginning of the healing process.

Topics

There is no standard format for subject matter in an ongoing group. Sometimes grandparents will talk about the system; sometimes they will talk about parenting issues, their own childhood, community resources, even their jobs. There is rarely an absence of topics. (However, Appendix B offers a list of common grandparenting issues for those moments when the discussion may run dry.)

Outreach

I do a lot of outreach work. I will spend months on the phone with a grandparent in crisis; sometimes I give one grandparent the phone number of another in a similar situation. Some will eventually come out for a meeting; others will just call to hear a supportive voice.

It can be difficult to get certain grandparents to attend a group, particularly in communities that have a strong emphasis on privacy and keeping problems in the family. If you have trouble with group attendance, plan a picnic for the kids. Grandparents may not make time to come out for themselves, but they will try harder for the children.

Kicking into High Gear

Once you have a cohesive group, there are a few other things you might want to try:

Outside Experts

I have found it beneficial to occasionally invite outside experts to address my groups. Attorneys, health care specialists, and representatives from the welfare department are among those who have been kind enough to attend our meetings and share their expertise. You might also ask a local mental health professional to conduct a series of parenting classes or invite someone who can demystify new technology—a lot has changed since you raised your first set of kids. But do not invite experts until your group has become a cohesive whole.

Family Activities

About once or twice a month, I plan a weekend activity that involves both grandparents and grandchildren. It is important for the children to realize that they are not alone; that many other kids are raised by grandparents; that "they're not the only ones with a Momma with gray hair," as one grandma puts it. Group activities raise everyone's morale. We frequently have potluck picnics at a local park, reserving a shelter area in advance to guarantee some shade. Events like these give kids space to run and allow grandparents time to relax and socialize with other adults. You might even consider inviting the parents occasionally, provided it's a healthy situation and the relationships are strong and positive.

Donated Tickets

Many families I work with are on fixed incomes, making it difficult to do the extras they would like to do for their grandchildren. I have, on occasion, been able to obtain donated group tickets to Disneyland, Barnum and Bailey Circus, the Ice Capades, Disney on Ice, local children's theaters, and various sporting events. Community organizations like the Junior League have hosted one-day events like a holiday gift-making party or a prom-prep event for the teens. Some summer camps have offered our kids discounted, and even free, tuition. We even had a special Mother's Day carnival, funded by an anonymous donor. And we've connected with other agencies that provide activities for relative caregivers. It takes lots of phone calls and letters (often just to find out who can make the decision to donate to a group). Don't get discouraged if you ask for something and get turned down. Just move on to the next request. Persistence generally does pay off.

Take Advantage of Group Pricing

All kinds of organizations offer group discounts, especially if the group is sizable. We have had grandparent families travel together, taking advantage of the camaraderie and the savings. One of our facilitators organized a trip to Laughlin, California, for 17 families—79 people in all. She was able to get inexpensive hotel rooms and a deal on vans. They attended a rodeo, saw the sites, enjoyed the pool, and traded off child care responsibilities, organizing activities for the kids while the adults rested or checked out the casinos—all on a very reasonable budget. Another year, a smaller group went to Las Vegas and the Grand Canyon. "Seeing all 31 kids laughing and running the trails and watching out for each other was amazing," she says.

Shared Skills

Your group is composed of grandparents who have diverse talents and abilities. You may decide to exchange these skills to help each other. For instance, in my groups I have grandparents who are willing to cut hair, repair appliances, fill out forms, and provide occasional respite care for other grandparents. One grandfather even provides a school shuttle for a grandmother who has no car. Another member owns a beauty salon and invited the whole group for a makeover day. Some grandparents have even volunteered to accompany each other to court. It can make you feel so much better to have someone there who cares, even when the outcome isn't positive. Exchange of these favors and services encourages mutual support.

Shared Goods

When good people come together, wonderful things happen, from clothing exchanges to acts of great generosity. Hand-me-downs were often easy pickings when you were young parents with friends who were also starting families. But when this second shift arrives late in life, you face childrearing alone—until you join a group.

One of the things my groups have organized is a clothing exchange. Grandparents bring in their grandchildren's outgrown clothing to share, and there are always families with younger grandchildren who are delighted to receive them. The same goes for toys, furniture, and other child accessories. If you do start something like this—and why not?—make sure that all donations are in good condition.

And then there is the magic . . .

When a grandfather in my group bought a new car, he and his wife donated their old one to a grandmother who didn't have one. When another grandmother could not afford to visit her dying brother, the group pooled its resources and came up with a round-trip ticket to send her to see him. One grandmother was mugged immediately after cashing the check to cover her rent and food; the grandparents came to her rescue with food and donations. And a few grandparents regularly help out several families with groceries. You can't plan or schedule magic like this, it just happens. But by keeping a group together, you do set the stage for great things.

Will Your Group Need a Mental Health Professional?

One of the things you need to consider when you set up your group is if you will need a mental health professional (that is, a social worker, psychologist, or counselor) and, if so, what his or her involvement will be.

A GAP group can work without a leader or therapist. You can become a big family, calling and supporting each other in times of stress. I have also trained facilitators to run groups, not just social workers but relative caregivers as well. You have to be really committed and it takes a long time, but if you know where to go when things get too intense, you may not need a regular mental health professional.

There are, however, situations that grandparent-facilitators cannot cope with on their own. At some point you may have a grandparent who is in a crisis that is beyond your capacity to handle. You could, for example, have a grandparent who is suicidal and needs to be hospitalized. As a fellow grandparent, you might not know where to start. Sometimes a grandparent or grandchild needs an outside referral or needs individual therapy in addition to a self-help group. Georgia Hill is a 49-year-old grandmother who has raised her grandson since her daughter died in a car accident four years ago. A recent car accident of her own jolted her back into the grieving process, opening up all kinds of old wounds. Georgia needs more intense therapy than a group alone can provide. I referred her to someone who specializes in bereavement counseling.

I would hate for any grandparent to give improper information to other grandparents about their grandchildren, adult children, or themselves. People don't intend to hurt each other, but they can—through lack of knowledge. For example, the line between discipline and child abuse is much thinner these days than when you were raising your own children, and a lot of grandparents are capable of unwittingly giving poor advice. Washing a child's mouth out with soap, for instance, used to be a perfectly acceptable way of punishing a foul mouth; by today's standards, it is considered abusive.

It can also destroy a group if someone gives the wrong information at a meeting and it backfires. It is always better to admit you don't know something and offer to try to find out. Write down such questions and find an outside resource.

This is where a mental health professional can be helpful. If you don't want a professional to facilitate your group, he or she can still be involved as a regular consultant, an on-call consultant, or a visiting expert. It's good to have someone on the sidelines who is available to consult on complicated issues. Perhaps he or she could attend the first few meetings, while your group is becoming cohesive. At the very least, I recommend having someone do a series of classes on parenting issues. You could even arrange a group for grandchildren, who also need to know they're not alone.

How to Find a Mental Health Professional

If you are in therapy or know another grandparent in therapy, talk to the therapist. He or she may be able to recommend someone. Perhaps a local counselor or social worker is already working with three or four grandparents. Check with your local child guidance or mental health clinic for referrals. Also, any place that does outpatient therapy is a good resource.

A Word to the Mental Health Professional

Years ago, I went on vacation and left another professional to fill in for me. She couldn't wait for me to return. "All I did was answer phone calls and deal with problems," she told me. "I didn't have time to do anything else." All she saw was a group of complaining, demanding old people. She was expecting it to be easy and got a real education. If you are a professional who is considering working with a GAP group, there are two questions you need to ask yourself: Do you have a special place in your heart for this population? Do you understand how these groups differ from traditional therapy groups?

When you work with a family in outpatient therapy, you work with their mental health needs, not with the washer breaking down and the car breaking down. You may see the children in outpatient therapy for an hour a week. Grandparent groups can be much more time consuming. We are dealing with whole families and many kinds of problems, and their needs are great. GAP groups deal with more than just emotional support. From the start, my philosophy has been that if you do not deal with basic needs, you cannot begin to deal with mental health needs.

When you work with traditional therapy groups, you have rules and commitments about time, frequency, and attendance. Grandparents may show up for a group meeting once a week or once in six months; they may pop in for half an hour between doctors' appointments or before a second-shift job. They are under incredible stress, and their own care is not their first priority. They may only come when they have a crisis, or they may call regularly for advice, feedback, suggestions, and resources. I have regular contact with a lot of grandparents I never see face to face but who call when they are in need.

You do end up giving more of yourself in a GAP group than in a traditional client–therapist relationship. But if you have a special feeling for grandparents, relative caregivers, nontraditional families, and their concerns, working with grandparent groups can be rewarding work.

GAP 2.0: ADVANCED SUPPORT AND THE ONE-STOP SHOP

Once a group has some experience under its belt, there are ways to expand the services you offer on several other levels, from immediate resources to advocacy and education programs. At GAP, we have grown into a one-stop shop for all the needs a grandparent or relative caregiver might encounter. If you have a core group of members who are out of crisis and able to volunteer time, you might consider expanding into some of the following areas:

Emergency Resources and Assistance

Many group facilitators keep a complete list of community resources and can refer caregivers to the right places to receive emergency food and clothing, emergency medical and dental services, even temporary shelter. GAP even has its own storage unit to save the things people donate today in preparation for a need tomorrow. For instance, I was at a meeting with a grandmother at the Department of Children and Family Services in Los Angeles. She was told that she had to have bedroom furniture for her five-year-old. We just happened to have a donated bedroom set on its way to storage that day. I made one phone call, and it was rerouted to her house by dinnertime.

Specialized Groups and Subgroups

A support group shows up in a community like a much-needed well. There is just one, and everyone comes to it for all their needs. But as you grow in experience and resources, including volunteers, you might want to build smaller, local wells that serve different purposes. Grandparents and relative caregivers have different needs depending on where they live, who they're raising, and, often, where they're from. You might consider offering a second group in a different neighborhood, or at a different time. In Los Angeles, for instance, it made sense to offer a group for Spanish speakers. We also have a group for grandparents raising teenagers and a children's group that meets concurrently with the adults so that the teens can express their own feelings in a safe and therapeutic environment. As you move into this stage, keep an eye out for subgroups that might benefit from their own meetings.

Community Outreach and Education

Your experience has value. Not just for your family, but for the families who will show up tomorrow, next week, and next year. So once the crisis has passed, you might find that relative caregivers will stay with the group in order to help others. That is certainly true for GAP. Often we train these volunteers to become group facilitators or to speak on behalf of the organization at community networking meetings. Several board members are relative caregivers who are also lawyers, business owners, or the heads of hospitals. A grandfather was our very first CEO, and an uncle is in charge of our storage and delivery. He picks up food at various churches and delivers it to families. Our members also staff an ongoing warm line that serves families and professionals across the United States, as well as a yearly conference. We try to use the talents of our volunteers in the best way possible, and it is their effort that keeps us growing.

GAP has also partnered with organizations like the Brookdale Foundation and the Child Welfare League of America to conduct workshops and presentations for grandparent groups, child welfare agencies, and government officials. We maintain a full-time office in the county children's court and developed a curriculum with the Children's Law Center for peer-to-peer counseling to help families navigate mental health services, the court system, and educational rights.

One of our newest outreach activities is our internship program. In the last few years, GAP has collaborated with various schools of social work and psychology to offer field training opportunities to undergraduate and master's students. They facilitate and co-facilitate our meetings, as well as helping out on various projects. Since some of the interns are already working for child welfare, they've given our relatives the experience of helping to educate social workers, while our interns have been sensitized to the issues, needs, and concerns of relative caregivers.

"We are trained to focus on child safety, and everything is quantity," says one intern. "Now I do my best to treat each individual as a human being instead of another case number."

"I've had grandparents in the past on my cases, but I treated them like normal foster parents," said another. "They're a unique population, and they definitely need more tender hands. Not because they're old and old-fashioned and don't get it, but because they are the children's family, and it's as devastating to the grandparents as to the parents. They need more kindness, more empathy, more understanding, more social work."

Of course, these programs developed slowly and over time. I point them out as a vision of what is possible. If your group is ready to move into community outreach, it doesn't have to be a huge leap. Can you invite social workers to get to know you? Is there an organization you could partner with where you can create respectful and mutually useful alliances? Start small, and see what opportunities unfold.

Advocacy

As your group grows in experience and reputation, you will find more and more ways to support grandparents in crisis. Advocacy is an immediate, practical way to help. GAP members have accompanied one another to meetings with child welfare workers, doctors, attorneys, and school administrators, and GAP has written letters on their behalf. For instance, Matt and Sophia Davis lost their grandson when they let their daughter stay for a night on her way to rehab. She didn't use in their house and was never alone with the baby, but when CPS found out, they took Donny and told the couple they would never get him back. We were able to arrange meetings and advocate on their behalf. Today not only do they have custody of Donny again, but they have adopted him. Of course, GAP has a 25 year history of working for the rights and concerns of caregiver-headed families. Through our community outreach, we have gained a reputation for being a strong, *informed* voice. As your group evolves, and as you do outreach, you may create important relationships that will serve your families in the future.

Activism

One person makes such a difference. A grandparent makes an enormous difference in the life of a neglected child. The person who starts a group helps each person who joins it. And one person joining forces with another person, and another, and another can change laws and move mountains. "The only way to make any changes in children's rights is for us to find each other and help each other," says Barbara Kirkland, founder of Grandparents Raising Grandchildren.[2]

There is strength in numbers, and in a digital age, those numbers can add up quickly. It is surprising how few e-mails, letters, or phone calls it takes to make legislators pay attention. It will not help a particular case—

those are still decided by individual judges—but it can change the next ones by creating awareness and political change.

Don't let the word *political* scare you. There are many ways to make a difference without actually speaking before the Senate or rallying on the Capitol steps—although some of our grandparents found those to be exciting experiences. You can work behind the scenes with legislators by sponsoring a bill, shaping a bill, or just supporting it with calls and e-mails. You can work with judges, attorneys, and social workers, offer them resources, and educate them about your concerns. You can work with the media and the community, creating public awareness and public education about children's rights and grandparents' rights.

For many caregivers, activism gives them a place to channel their anger and their energy. "You feel like you're doing something," one grandmother explains. "You're not sitting and wallowing in your pain." "This has become a passion with me," says another. "I want to be a part of helping these children have a voice, with education, changing laws, whatever it takes."

If that kind of activism calls to you, or your group, try to connect with organizations that are already working to impact policy. They will be able to help you navigate the process, identify the players, and make the best use of the tools available to you.

Evolving into Family

You just can't help it. You can't spend all this time discussing family, helping each other's families, watching your grandchildren play together, and helping each other in times of need without becoming a kind of ad hoc family yourselves. I know grandkids who, when told they have plans with family, will ask, "Our family or GAP family?" And in some cases, GAP is the better answer, the bringer of smiles. The reasons aren't hard to understand. As common as it is for grandparents to raise their grandchildren today (not to mention great-grandparents, aunts, uncles, cousins, and siblings), it's still not the way the world expects families to look. At GAP events, all the kids are being raised by relatives, and all the adults understand the issues the others are facing. There is great comfort in that.

Nor do all caregivers have access to their own families. Their people may be far away or dead, in jail or just missing. In some cases, they may have even cut them off. That's what happened to Marta Ramirez. She has ten children, but none will visit her since she took in her grandsons. GAP, for her, means that people call and ask how she's feeling, how her day went. It means that the boys have regular picnics and parties with people who may not be connected by birth but who, over time, have become surrogate cousins, aunts, and uncles.

"GAP gave me family," another grandmother agrees. "It gave me something I could trust. It gave me a place where I wasn't an alien. I wasn't weird. I wasn't different. I was just somebody doing the best I could."

It's not something you can plan for, manage, or orchestrate. But when you consistently create safe, nurturing space, amazing things can happen. And not only between families.

A Speaking Heart

Jessica Hernandez was one of our wonderful interns. A caseworker and child abuse investigator by day and a master's student in social work at night, she helped to co-facilitate our Spanish-speaking groups. Toward the end of her internship, she had to make a class presentation on her experience. It came out as a poem, written in the voice of the relative caregivers themselves, and based on the Mexican folk legend of La Llorona, a ghostly woman who wanders the night, calling out for her lost children. I could not have imagined, 25 years ago, that a social worker could understand and respect the feelings of our population so completely. I include it here, with Jessica's permission, as a reminder of what is possible when we join together with open hearts for support, education, and advocacy (a full English version is in Appendix C).

Gracias to the Relatives of La Llorona
by Jessica Hernandez[3]

Abuelos, tías, uncles
Names that I could only hear in an echo
I was suddenly stripped away from my role
Because abuse, drogas, jail, and la muerte became the new children of my
     hijos
And like La Llorona, I was caught in her canto
Saying, "Ay mis hijos, ay mis hijos."

I felt lost, guilt, shame, anger, and sadness
I cried and cried each night with La Llorona in perfect harmony
"Ay mis hijos, ay mis hijos"
While searching for the gates of a community that would help me re-parent
I wanted my nietos, nieces, y sobrinos to know that I, too,
Nourished, respected, and loved them (as I once did their parents)
I needed community to let me know that I am not alone
Searching each day for the right song
So that today I can say with love, respect, y orgullo, "Si, son mis hijos."
La Llorona is not taking them!
And before I go to bed tonight, I'll silently say a prayer for mom and dad
Who drowned at La Llorona's waters.
Because I still hear my name in the echo
Abuelos, tías, uncles
This is for you. . . .
Gracias for not letting me drown!

15

Conclusion

You know they say blood is thicker than water? Well, for us, love is thicker than blood.
　　　　　　　　—Jonathan Williams, 37, raised by stepgrandmother
　　　　　　　　　　and grandfather[1]

Years ago, grandmother and grandparent advocate Ethel Dunn wrote a moving article about Las Madres de la Plaza de Mayo (the mothers of the Plaza de Mayo). These were the middle- and upper-class mothers and grandmothers of Argentina who gathered each Thursday in the square outside Argentina's White House to protest the disappearance of thousands of children and grandchildren during the military government's campaign against "subversives" in the mid-1970s and early 1980s. As many as 4,000 of these children were believed to have been kidnapped and turned over to military families for adoption. These grieving mothers and grandmothers translated their fear into anger and their anger into advocacy; they walked in a large silent circle, week after week, carrying pictures of missing children. It is a story of courage, love, and determination.

In our own country there is no military government spiriting away children. But since the 1980s, drugs and alcohol, violent crime, child abuse, and bureaucratic red tape have endangered far more than 4,000 children. Here, too, thousands of grandparents are turning grief and fear into action and advocacy. "Sometimes we, too, march, picket, carry signs, and demand," wrote Dunn. "We never stop trying to educate. We sometimes become angry, often frustrated. Once in a while we smell the passionate fragrance of success and allow ourselves a short period of time to rejoice. Always, however, we persevere."[2]

Persevere. It means to continue in spite of difficulty and opposition. It doesn't matter if you are on a picket line or in a grocery line; every grandparent trying to raise a grandchild perseveres. Each morning your grandchildren wake up safe and each night they go to bed well loved and well cared for, you have succeeded. Each grandparent who has lost a grandchild perseveres, and each day that grandparent survives the sorrow, he or she has succeeded.

Grandparents in Los Angeles, California, and Paducah, Kentucky, have as much to tell about courage, love, and determination as Las Madres de la Plaza de Mayo. If you ever wonder where the rewards come from, consider the following letter, which was written by my nephew Kevin when he was in college.[3] It was addressed to my mother, the grandmother who raised him:

Nona,

On July 31st, 1983, you unexpectedly became a mother again. You took an 8-year-old boy into your home and treated him like he was your son, as if it was normal.

Your life was turned upside down. You lost the most precious thing in the world to you—your daughter. In the middle of your pain and suffering you found the time to take care of a scared, confused, and uncertain little boy who had just lost his mother.

As the little boy got older, he learned how to push your buttons. He had a knack for making your day miserable. Making life hard for you was his way of saying he didn't want another mom. He did everything he could to push you away, but you wouldn't leave him alone. The more problems he caused, the more you were there for him—getting him out of trouble and pushing him to do something with his life. You never thought twice about helping him when he needed it. When he was sick, you nursed him back to health.

When he wanted a ride to a friend's house, you took him there. You always tried your hardest to make him happy.

Now he has grown up and understands the sacrifices you made for him.

Nona, this little boy is a very grateful young man now, and I want you to know how much I appreciate all you've done for me.

I want you to know that I'm proud to be your grandson. But most of all, I want you to know I love you.

Kevin

The great American poet Carl Sandburg once said, "A baby is God's opinion that the world should go on."[4] When you take in a grandchild, you do more than help one family; you preserve our future.

Appendices

Appendix A
Resources for Grandparents and Relative Caregivers

TO CONTACT SYLVIE OR GAP

Grandparents As Parents (GAP)
Website: *www.grandparentsasparents.org*
E-mail: sylvie@grandparentsasparents.org
Office phone: (818) 264-0880
Office fax: (818) 264-0882
Sylvie: (818) 789-1177
Mailing address:
22048 Sherman Way #217
Canoga Park, CA 91303

FOR FINDING GROUPS IN YOUR AREA

AARP Foundation GrandCare Support Locator
Website: *www.aarp.org/families/grandparents/gic*
E-mail: gic@aarp.org
Toll-free: (888) OUR-AARP (888-687-2277)

Brookdale Foundation
Website: *www.brookdalefoundation.org*
Phone: (212) 308-7355

Brookdale's Relatives as Parents Program (RAPP) was established in 1996 to promote the creation or expansion of services for grandparents and relative caregivers. They host an annual conference and offer a listserv, site bulletins, Web chats, and a newsletter.

Generations United

Website: *www.gu.org*

Phone: (202) 289-3979

A national membership organization that works to improve the lives of children, youth, and older people through intergenerational strategies, programs, and public policies.

Grandfamilies of America

Website: *www.grandfamiliesofamerica.com*

Phone: (301) 358-3911

National Committee of Grandparents for Children's Rights

Website: *www.grandparentsforchildren.org*

Phone: (518) 833-0215

A nationwide network of grandparents, community members, and professionals working to provide education, support, and advocacy for children, grandparents, and kinship families.

SOURCES OF ADDITIONAL SUPPORT

Al-Anon (also Alateen and Alatot)

In the United States and Canada:

Website: *www.al-anon.alateen.org*

You can also look up Al-Anon in your telephone book for information on local groups.

Compassionate Friends

Website: *www.compassionatefriends.org*

Toll-free: (877) 969-0010; (630) 990-0010

A group for bereaved parents who have lost children of any age, for any reason.

Our House

Website: *www.ourhouse-grief.org*

A grief support center based in Los Angeles. The Resources section of their website has a book list for children and teens.

PARENTING AND EDUCATION RESOURCES

American Council for Drug Education
Website: *www.acde.org*

Children and Adults with Attention Deficit/Hyperactivity Disorder (CHADD)
Website: *www.chadd.org*
Toll-free: (800) 233-4050; (301) 306-7070

Learning Disabilities Association (LDA)
Website: *www.ldaamerica.org*
Phone: (412) 341-1515
    An association for children and adults with learning disabilities.

MyCarePack
Website: *http://mycarepack.com/index.aspx*
    A national service to help families securely send care packages directly to an incarcerated family member.

National Alliance on Mental Illness (NAMI)
Website: *www.nami.org*
Toll free: 800-950-NAMI

National Disability Rights Network
Website: *www.napas.org*
    Provides information on protection and advocacy for individuals with disabilities.

National Information Center for Children and Youth with Disabilities (NICHCY)
Website: *www.nichcy.org*
Website in Spanish: *www.nichcy.org/espanol*
Toll-free: (800) 695-0285
    A national information center that provides information on disabilities and disability-related issues, focusing on children and youth, from birth to age 22. NICHCY publications include explanations of special education laws and school

services for children with disabilities, state resource sheets, and information on individual disabilities. They also offer State Resource Sheets to help you connect with disability agencies and organizations in your state.

National Institute on Drug Abuse (NIDA)

Website: *www.drugabuse.gov*

   NIDA provides drug information and a counseling hotline.

Wrightslaw

Website: *www.wrightslaw.com*

   A central information center for information about special education law, education law, and advocacy for children with disabilities.

GOVERNMENT ASSISTANCE RESOURCES

Child Welfare Information Gateway

Website: *www.childwelfare.gov*

   A service of the Children's Bureau, Administration for Children and Families, U.S. Department of Health and Human Services. It provides access to information on child welfare and neglect, out-of-home care, adoption, and more through websites, databases, print and electronic publications, and other online learning tools. The site includes links to state-specific resources, including the Adoption Assistance by State Database at *www.childwelfare.gov/adoption/adopt_assistance*.

Kinship Navigator Programs

   These are state initiatives (partially funded by federal grants) that provide referrals, information, and follow-up services to relative caregivers to connect them with benefits and services that they or the children need. Google "kinship navigator program" and your state for a program near you.

North American Council on Adoptable Children (NACAC)

Website: *www.nacac.org*

Toll-free: (800) 470-6665

   An organization that supports foster, adoptive, and kinship families through information, referral, and advocacy. They have comprehensive information on AAP, adoption tax credit, support groups, and postadoption programs throughout the United States. For current information on the adoption tax credit, go to *www.nacac.org/taxcredit/taxcredit.html*.

Appendix B
Conversation Topics for Grandparent Support Groups

THE STORIES

- How many grandchildren you have and how you came to have them.

LIFE CHANGES

- The impact on your social life now that you're a parent again.
- How your life is different from those of your friends.
- How your grandchildren have changed your work life.
- Your feelings about work.
- The financial strain of raising a second family.
- The dreams and plans that have been put on hold.
- The toll on your health.

INTENSE FEELINGS

- Grief over the loss of your adult child.
- Anger at your adult child, the situation, the system, everything.
- Guilt.

- Depression.
- Feeling you don't want to raise your grandchildren, but not wanting them split up or placed with strangers.
- Feeling you don't belong anywhere, neither with young parents nor with adults your age.
- Fears.
- Hopes for your grandchildren.
- When and how to seek outside therapy for yourself as an individual or a couple.

PARENTING ISSUES

- Changes in childrearing techniques since you brought up your own kids.
- The effects of the parent's visits on the child's behavior and emotions.
- Dealing with school problems children might have.
- Setting limits with grandchildren and adult children; what behaviors you will or will not tolerate.
- Recognizing age-appropriate behavior.
- Setting age-appropriate consequences.
- How to raise your grandchild's self-esteem.
- How to help children who were born drug exposed.
- Learning to accept that some grandchildren might need more help than you can provide.
- When and how to seek outside therapy for your grandchildren.

YOUR ADULT CHILDREN

- Learning to accept the fact that your son or daughter is choosing to be an irresponsible parent.
- How to set appropriate boundaries with your adult child.
- When to decide that you have done enough for your adult child and that it's time to let go.
- Deciding whether or not to maintain contact with an adult child in jail.
- Protecting yourself and your grandchildren from your adult child.
- When and how to consider reconnecting with your adult child and reestablishing trust.

THE REST OF YOUR FAMILY

- The reaction of other children and family members to your becoming a parent again.
- Handling sibling rivalry.
- The effects of second parenthood on your marriage.

THE BUREAUCRACY

- How to negotiate the bureaucracy of government agencies.
- How to decipher the language and rules of the juvenile dependency system.
- Handling the feelings that come up around bureaucratic roadblocks.
- How to navigate the challenges of the school system and special education.

Appendix C

Thank You to the Relatives of The Crying Woman

(ENGLISH TRANSLATION)

by Jessica Hernandez

Grandfathers, aunts, uncles
Names that I could only hear in an echo
I was suddenly stripped away from my role
Because abuse, drugs, jail, and death became the new children of my children
And like The Crying Woman, I was caught in her song
Saying, "Ay my children, ah my children."
I felt lost, guilt, shame, anger, and sadness
I cried and cried each night with The Crying Woman in perfect harmony
"Ah my children, ah my children."
While searching for the gates of a community that would help me re-parent
I wanted my grandchildren, nieces, and nephews to know that I, too,
Nourished, respected, and loved them (as I once did their parents)
I needed community to let me know that I am not alone
Searching each day for the right song
So that today I can say with love, respect, and pride, "Yes, these are my children."
The Crying Woman is not taking them!

And before I go to bed tonight, I'll silently say a prayer for mom and dad
Who drowned at The Crying Woman's waters.
Because I still hear my name in the echo
Grandfathers, aunts, uncles
This is for you . . .
Thank you for not letting me drown!

Notes

PREFACE

1. When we wrote the first edition, the number of children born with drugs in their system each year was at 375,000. By 2010, that number had grown to somewhere between 550,000 and 750,000, and may not include babies exposed to prescription drugs. Richard Martin. "Prescription drug epidemic spreads to babies," *St. Petersburg Times* (now *Tampa Bay Times*), July 18, 2010. Available at *www.tampabay.com/news/health/article1109848.ece*.

2. The number of child deaths per day due to child abuse and neglect doubled between 1995 and 2007. The real statistics might be higher, as the true cause of 50 to 60 percent of child fatalities may not be recorded on the death certificate. ChildHelp. *National Child Abuse Statistics*, accessed May 25, 2012. Available at *www.childhelp.org/pages/statistics*.

3. The actual percentage of inmates who are parents is down, from 80 percent to 50 percent, but that is only because the prison population itself has grown so much. The Sentencing Project. *Incarcerated Parents and Their Children: Trends 1991–2007*. Washington, DC: The Sentencing Project, February 2009.

INTRODUCTION

1. Linda L. Creighton. "Silent Saviors," *U.S. News & World Report*, December 16, 1991, p. 83.

2. Mary Lou Wilson. "Recycled Parents," *The Reporter* (Vacaville, California), March 19, 1990, p. 1A.

3. Andrew H. Malcolm. "Helping Grandparents Who Are Parents Again," *The New York Times,* November 19, 1991. Available at *www.nytimes.com/1991/11/19/ nyregion/our-towns-helping-grandparents-who-are-parents-again.html.*

4. Lenora Madison Poe. *Black Grandparents as Parents.* Berkeley, CA: Lenora Madison Poe, 1992; Meredith Minkler and Kathleen M. Roe. *Grandmothers as Caregivers: Raising Children of the Crack Cocaine Epidemic.* Newbury Park, CA: Sage Publications, 1993; Irene M. Endicott. *Grandparenting Redefined: Guidance for Today's Changing Family.* Lynwood, WA: Aglow Publications, 1992.

CHAPTER 1

1. Jill Smolowe. "To Grandma's House We Go," *Time,* November 5, 1990, p. 90.

2. Ibid., p. 86; Meredith Minkler and Kathleen M. Roe. *Grandmothers as Caregivers: Raising Children of the Crack Cocaine Epidemic.* Newbury Park, CA: Sage Publications, 1993, pp. x, 4–5.

3. Rose M. Kreider and Renee Ellis. "Living Arrangements of Children: 2009," *Current Population Reports,* P70-126. Washington, DC: U.S. Census Bureau, 2011.

4. Ibid.

5. Mike Yorkey. "Picking Up the Pieces," *Focus on the Family,* September 1993, p. 13.

6. Leadership Council on Child Abuse and Interpersonal Violence. "How Many Children Are Court-Ordered into Unsupervised Contact with an Abusive Parent after Divorce?" Baltimore, MD: Leadership Council on Child Abuse and Interpersonal Violence, September 22, 2008 (press release).

7. Guttmacher Institute. *Facts on American Teens' Sexual and Reproductive Health.* Washington, DC: Guttmacher Institute, accessed February 2012. Available at *www.guttmacher.org/pubs/FB-ATSRH.html.*

8. Annie E. Casey Foundation. *Kids Count Data Book: State Profiles of Child Well-Being.* Washington, DC: Annie E. Casey Foundation, 2010, p. 26.

9. ChildHelp. *National Child Abuse Statistics,* accessed May 25, 2012. Available at *www.childhelp.org/pages/statistics.*

10. Lauren E. Glaze and Laura M. Maruschak. *Parents in Prison and Their Minor Children,* cited in *An Estimated 809,800 Inmates in the Nation's Prisons Were Parents to 1,706,600 Minor Children at Midyear 2007,* August 26, 2008. Washington, DC: Bureau of Justice Statistics (press release).

11. Richard Martin. "Prescription drug epidemic spreads to babies," *St. Petersburg Times* (now *Tampa Bay Times*), July 18, 2010. Available at *www.tampabay.com/news/health/article1109348.ece.*

12. Johns Hopkins Medical Children's Center. "Children Who Lose a Parent to Suicide More Likely to Die the Same Way." Baltimore, MD: Johns Hopkins Medical Children's Center, April 21, 2010 (press release).
13. Marqueece Harris-Dawson. "For Grandparents Day, let's support the care they give," *The Sacramento Bee*, September 9, 2011.
14. Interview with Dr. Michael Jones, marriage and family therapist, by authors (via telephone), Newport Beach, California, June 22, 1994.

CHAPTER 3

1. Andrew H. Malcolm. "Helping Grandparents Who Are Parents Again," *The New York Times*, November 19, 1991. Available at *www.nytimes.com/1991/11/19/nyregion/our-towns-helping-grandparents-who-are-parents-again.html*.
2. *Donahue*. April 11, 1991.
3. Susan R. Pollack. "The Grandparent Trap," *The Detroit News*, July 17, 1991, p. 1C.
4. Tony Link. "When Kids Come to Grandma's House to Stay," *Daily News* (Los Angeles), December 19, 1989, p. 3.
5. Laura Accinelli. "Starting Over," *Daily Breeze* (Torrance, California), September 11, 1988, p. D1.
6. Madeleine Wild. "Grandmas Forced to Become Moms," *Woman's World*, July 16, 1991, p. 21.

CHAPTER 4

1. Eileen Beal. "Grandparents Raising Grandchildren," *Cleveland Jewish News*, November 23, 1990, p. 15.

CHAPTER 5

1. *Seniors Speak Out*, KPBS TV, San Diego, November 26, 1992.
2. Muriel Dobbin. "Grandmothers Fill In for Drug-Abusing Parents," *Senior Highlights*, March 1990, p. 5.
3. Harriet Goldhor Lerner. *The Dance of Intimacy*. New York: Harper & Row, 1989, p. 27.
4. Correspondence with Mary Weaver, executive director, Friends Outside, Los Angeles, California, October 5, 2011.

CHAPTER 6

1. Robin Worthington. "The Second Time Around," *San Jose Mercury News,* March 22, 1992, p. 51.
2. Sherry Angel. "Starting Over: Grandparents Who Step In and Raise Their Grandchildren," *Los Angeles Times/Orange County,* April 15, 1991, p. E3.
3. Ingrid Watson. "Rocking the Cradle," *Fort Worth Star-Telegram,* November 13, 1988, p. 7.
4. Annie E. Casey Foundation. *Kids Count Data Book: State Profiles of Child Well-Being.* Washington, DC: Annie E. Casey Foundation, 2010, p. 26.
5. Interview with Dr. Gigi L. Johnson, executive director, Maremel Institute, by authors (via telephone), Monrovia, California, August 24, 2011.
6. Correspondence with Dr. Gigi L. Johnson, executive director, Maremel Institute, Monrovia, California, January 4, 2012.
7. Ibid.
8. For a full definition of ADHD, see American Psychiatric Association. *Diagnostic and Statistical Manual of Mental Disorders,* (4th ed., text revision). Washington, DC: American Psychiatric Association, 2000, pp. 86–93.
9. Christine S. Moyer. "ADHD Rises 32% among Children and Teens," *American Medical News,* September 2, 2011. Available at *www.ama-assn.org/amednews/2011/08/29/hlsb0902.htm.*
10. U.S. Department of Health and Human Services. *Mental Health: A Report of the Surgeon General.* Rockville, MD: U.S. Department of Health and Human Services, Substance Abuse and Mental Health Services Administration, Center for Mental Health Services, National Institutes of Health, National Institute of Mental Health, 1999, Chapter 3. Available at *http://137.187.25.243/library/mentalhealth/chapter3/sec4.html.*
11. American Psychiatric Association. *Diagnostic and Statistical Manual,* pp. 86–93.
12. Eileen Mayers Pasztor, Donna D. Petras, & Cassaundra Rainey. *Collaborating with Kinship Caregivers: A Research to Practice, Competency-Based Training Program for Child Welfare Workers and Their Supervisors.* Washington, DC: Child Welfare League of America, 2012.
13. Jane Glenn Haas. "It Can Be Grand to Be Raised by Grandparents," *The Orange County Register,* March 25, 1992. Available in the archives at *www.ocregister.com/articles/archives-218862-county-orange.html.*

CHAPTER 7

1. National Information Center for Children and Youth with Disabilities. *Learning Disabilities* (Fact Sheet Number 7. Washington, DC: National Information

Center for Children and Youth with Disabilities, 2011; Centers for Disease Control and Prevention. *Attention Deficit/Hyperactivity Disorder (ADHD): Data & Statistics.* Washington, DC: Centers for Disease Control and Prevention, 2010. Available at *www.cdc.gov/ncbddd/adhd/data.html.*

2. "Eight Famous Persons with Learning Disabilities," *Their World*, January 1981, p. 67.

CHAPTER 8

1. Muriel Dobbins. "Grandmothers Fill In for Drug-Abusing Parents," *Senior Highlights*, March 1990, p. 5.

2. JoBeth McDaniel. "The Second Shift," *Life*, June 1, 1992, p. 65.

3. Lisa Girion, Scott Glover, and Doug Smith. "Drug Deaths Now Outnumber Traffic Fatalities in U.S., Data Show," *Los Angeles Times*, September 17, 2011. Available at *http://articles.latimes.com/zou/sep/17/local/la-me-drugs-epidemic-20110918.*

4. Centers for Disease Control and Prevention. "Prescription Painkiller Overdoses at Epidemic Levels: Kill More Americans than Heroin and Cocaine Combined." Atlanta, GA: Centers for Disease Control and Prevention, November 1, 2011 (press release).

5. "Study: 22 Million Americans Use Illegal Drugs," *CNN Health*, September 8, 2011. Available at *http://thechart.blogs.cnn.com/2011/09/08/study-22-million-americans-use-illegal-drugs-3.*

6. McDaniel. "Second Shift," p. 66.

7. U.S. Senate Committee on Labor and Human Resources, Subcommittee on Children, Family, Drugs, and Alcoholism. *Falling through the Crack: The Impact of Drug-Exposed Children on the Child Welfare System* (March 8, 1990). Washington, DC: U.S. Government Printing Office, 1990, p. 58.

8. Ibid., p. 164.

9. *Donahue*, April 11, 1991.

10. Interview with Jacqueline Battle, Infants of Substance Abusing Mothers, Los Angeles County–University of Southern California Medical Center, by authors, Los Angeles, California, October 1, 1993.

11. Interview with Dorsey Nunn, Legal Services for Prisoners with Children, by authors, Los Angeles, California, November 4, 1993.

12. National Center on Substance Abuse and Child Welfare. *Substance-Exposed Infants*, accessed March 2012. Available at *www.ncsacw.samhsa.gov/resources/substance-exposed-infants.aspx.*

13. Guttmacher Institute. *Substance Abuse during Pregnancy, State Policies in Brief, 2012*, accessed May 1, 2012. Available at *www.guttmacher.org/statecenter/spibs/spib_SADP.pdf.*

14. Gateway Recovery Services and the Pathology Department of Borgess Hospital. *Drugs of Abuse Information Sheet.* Available at *www.ncsconline.org/wc/publications/res_judedu_substanceabusematerial19pub.pdf.*
15. Anastasia Toufexis. "Innocent Victims," *Time,* May 13, 1991, p. 59.
16. Interview with Fay Strassburger, California grandmother, by authors, Los Angeles, California, May 18, 1994.
17. Melissa Balmain Welner. "A Testament to Survival," *Orange County Register,* June 14, 1992.
18. Judy Lin. "Recruit in War on Drugs Has Own Battle Scars," *Los Angeles Times,* March 22, 1999. Available at *http://articles.latimes.com/1999/mar/22/local/me-19822*; "President Names Members to the Commission on Drug Free Communities." Washington, DC: Office of the Press Secretary, October 30, 1998 (press release).
19. Alice Park. "Teens and Drugs: Rite of Passage or Recipe for Addiction?" *Time,* June 29, 2011. Available at *www.healthland.time.com.*
20. Superintendent of Documents, U.S. Government Printing Office. *The Abuse of Prescription and Over-the-Counter Drugs.* Available at *http://theantidrug.com/pdfs/resources/teen-rx/Prescription_Abuse_brochure.pdf.*

CHAPTER 10

1. "Family 'Kin Care' Trend Increasing," *NASW News,* May 1992.
2. Ingrid Watson. "Rocking the Cradle," *Fort Worth Star-Telegram,* November 13, 1988, p. 6.
3. Trish Johnson. "'Older' Parents Need Support," *Katy Times,* February 25, 1990, p. 3A.
4. Correspondence with attorney Joseph MacKenzie by authors, Los Angeles, California, December 23, 2010, and May 29, 2012.
5. Interview with attorney Joseph MacKenzie by authors, Los Angeles, California, December 20, 2010; correspondence with attorney Joseph MacKenzie by authors, Los Angeles, California, May 29, 2012.
6. Susan Swartz. "When Grandparents Are Parents Again," *Press Democrat* (Santa Rosa, California), July 14, 1991, p. D1.
7. Interview with Harold LaFlamme, California attorney, by authors, Buena Park, California, February 20, 1993.
8. Ibid.
9. Legal guardianship ends at age 18 in California; your state may differ.
10. Chicago Legal Advocacy for Incarcerated Mothers. "When a Parent is Arrested: Caring for the Children." Chicago, IL: Chicago Legal Advocacy for Incarcerated Mothers, 2009, p. 5.

11. Judicial Council of California. *Guardianship Pamphlet*, JV-350 (New July 1, 1989), p. 4.

12. Interview with Robert Walmsley, California attorney, by authors, Buena Park, California, February 20, 1993.

13. Child Welfare Information Gateway. *Consent to Adoption*. Washington, DC: U.S. Department of Health and Human Services, Children's Bureau, 2010.

14. Fran H. Zupan. "Love is Grand," *State Newspaper* (Columbia, South Carolina), April 9, 1992, p. 4D.

CHAPTER 11

1. Interview with Ted Youmans, California attorney, by authors, Santa Ana, California, March 6, 1993.

2. Correspondence with Marjorie Shelvy, senior attorney, Legal Aid Foundation of Los Angeles, May 13, 2010.

3. Interview with Leslie Starr Heimov, executive director, Children's Law Center of California, by authors (via telephone), April 27, 2012.

4. The petition of dependency must be filed within 48 hours in California. California Welfare and Institutions Code Sections, accessed October 25, 2012. Available at *http://law.onecle.com/california/welfare/313.html*.

5. Telephone interview with Leslie Starr Heimov, by authors, April 27, 2012.

6. Correspondence with Leslie Starr Heimov, executive director, Children's Law Center of California, October 24, 2012.

7. Children's Law Center of Los Angeles. *Grandparents as Parents Relative Caregiver Training Manual*. Los Angeles, CA: Children's Law Center of Los Angeles, 2010.

8. Interview with Pamela Mohr, former executive director, Alliance for Children's Rights, by authors, Los Angeles, California, February 24, 1993.

9. Correspondence with Leslie Starr Heimov, executive director, Children's Law Center of California, October 24, 2012.

10. Interview with Leslie Heimov, op cit.

11. Interview with Leslie Heimov, executive director, Children's Law Center of California, by authors (via telephone), April 27, 2012.

12. Interview with Ted Youmans, by authors, March 6, 1993.

13. Ellen Palmer. "Grandparents Raising Grandchildren—The Golden Years: Cancelled," *Valley Magazine* (Orange County Beach Cities, California), December 1990, p. 11.

14. U.S. Senate Committee on Labor and Human Resources. *Falling through the Crack: The Impact of Drug-Exposed Children on the Child Welfare System* (March 8, 1990). Washington, DC: U.S. Government Printing Office, 1990, p. 58.

15. Interview with Ethel Dunn, executive director, Grandparents United for Children's Rights, by authors (via telephone), September 19, 1993.

16. Interview with Charles Ollinger, Arizona attorney, by authors, Long Beach, California, October 22, 1993.

17. Legal Services for Prisoners with Children. *Manual for Grandparent-Relative Caregivers and Their Advocates* (3rd ed.), San Francisco, CA: Legal Services for Prisoners with Children, 2002, p. 1.

18. Interview with John C. Wooley, California judge, by authors, Buena Park, California, February 20, 1993.

CHAPTER 12

1. U.S. House of Representatives Committee on Ways and Means. *2008 Green Book*. Washington, DC: Author. Table 11-15, pp. 56–58, accessed October 19, 2012. Available at *http://waysandmeans.house.gov/media/pdf/111/s111cw.pdf.*

2. U.S. House of Representatives Committee on Ways and Means. *2011 Green Book*. Washington, DC: Author. Table 7-23, accessed October 19, 2012. Available at *http://greenbook.waysandmeans.house.gov.*

3. Correspondence with Marjorie Shelvy, senior attorney, Legal Aid Foundation of Los Angeles, May 16, 2012.

4. Foster care benefits are defined in Title IV-E of the Social Security Act, 42 U.S.C. 670 et seq., and are known as IV-E Foster Care.

5. Daniel Heimpel, "Children of the System," *The Daily Beast/Newsweek*, March 8, 2009. See also 89.3KPCC (Southern California Public Radio), October 1, 2010. "The Power of 3 Extra Years: AB12 to the Rescued California Foster Youth." Available at *www.scpr.org/programs/patt-morrison/2010/10/01/16285/ab12-signed.*

6. Jeffrey Miller. "Woman Fights Social Service Agencies," *Los Angeles Times*, January 3, 1988.

7. Social Security Administration. *Benefits for Children with Disabilities*. Baltimore, MD: Social Security Administration, 2011, p. 7.

8. Ibid.

9. Social Security Administration. *Benefits for Children with Disabilities,* p. 8.

10. Social Security Administration. *Survivors Benefits* (SSA Pub. No. 05-10084). Baltimore, MD: Social Security Administration, April 2011, p. 4.

11. Correspondence with Josh Kroll, project coordinator of the Adoption Subsidy Resource Center of the North American Council on Adoptable Children (NACAC), June 1, 2012.

12. Ibid.

13. Center for Law and Social Policy and Children's Defense Fund, together with

16 collaborating national organizations. *New Help for Children Raised by Grandparents and Other Relatives: Questions and Answers about the Fostering Connections to Success and Increasing Adoptions Act of 2008,* January 2009, Section 4.33, p. 46. Available at *www.childrensdefense.org* under Research Library.

14. 42 U.S.C. § 1396d(r)(5) of the Medicaid Act. Cited in Jane Perkins. *Advocate's Medicaid EPSDT Reference Manual.* Chapel Hill, NC: National Health Law Program, 1993, p. 21.

CHAPTER 13

1. Attributed to Walter Barbee. Source unknown.

2. "Legal Rights Because of Learning Disabilities," *L/D Law,* 1990, p. 13.

3. Ibid., p. 13.

4. Rehabilitation Act of 1973. 29 U.S.C. 794 et seq., § 504, as explained in "Legal Rights Because of Learning Disabilities," p. 13.

5. The reauthorized Individuals with Disabilities Education Act was signed into law on December 3, 2004. It can be found in Volume 20 of the United States Code (U.S.C.) beginning at Section 1400. 20 U.S.C. § 1400(d).

6. Interview with Larry Hanna, California attorney and former special education commissioner for the Los Angeles Unified School District, by authors, Los Angeles, California, May 13, 1993.

7. Correspondence with Pamela Darr Wright of *www.wrightslaw,* May 7, 2012.

8. Ibid.

9. Interview with Jill Rowland, Director of Special Education Programs, Alliance for Children's Rights, by authors (via telephone), May 2011.

10. Interview with Larry Hanna by authors, May 13, 1993.

CHAPTER 14

1. Warren Harris. "Raising Second Family," *Las Vegas Sun,* June 19, 1989, p. 1B.

2. Patty Housen. "Retiring to the Nursery: Grandparents Raising Kids' Kids," *Senior Beacon: In Focus for People over 50,* May 1990, p. 1.

3. Jessica Hernandez. "Gracias to the Relatives of La Llorona." *Grandparents As Parents: Filling the Gap,* Summer 2012, p. 4.

CHAPTER 15

1. Alice Hornbaker. "Parents Second Time Around," *Cincinnati Enquirer,* September 10, 1991, p. 2.

2. Ethel Dunn. "Those Wonderful Abuelas," *Intergenerational Hookup*, Winter/
   Spring 1993, p. 1.
3. Reprinted with permission of Kevin de Toledo.
4. Donald O. Bolander, Dolores D. Varner, Gary B. Wright, and Stephanie H.
   Greene (compilers). *Instant Quotation Dictionary*. Little Falls, NJ: Career Publishing, 1981, p. 30.

Bibliography

BOOKS/MANUALS/HEARINGS

American Psychiatric Association. *Diagnostic and Statistical Manual of Mental Disorders,* (4th ed., text revision). Washington, DC: American Psychiatric Association, 2000.

Annie E. Casey Foundation. *Kids Count Data Book: State Profiles of Child Well-Being.* Washington, DC: Annie E. Casey Foundation, 2010.

Bolander, Donald O., Dolores D. Varner, Gary B. Wright, and Stephanie H. Greene (compilers). *Instant Quotation Dictionary.* Little Falls, NJ: Career Publishing, 1981.

Children's Law Center of Los Angeles. *Grandparents as Parents Relative Caregiver Training Manual.* Los Angeles, CA: Children's Law Center of Los Angeles, 2010.

Endicott, Irene M. *Grandparenting Redefined: Guidance for Today's Changing Family.* Lynwood, WA: Aglow Publications, 1992.

Keller, Helen. *We Bereaved.* New York: Leslie Fulenwider, 1929.

Kreider, Rose M., and Renee Ellis. "Living Arrangements of Children: 2009," *Current Population Reports,* P70-126. Washington, DC: U.S. Census Bureau, 2011.

Legal Services for Prisoners with Children. *Manual for Grandparent-Relative Caregivers and Their Advocates* (3rd ed.). San Francisco, CA: Legal Services for Prisoners with Children, 2002.

Lerner, Harriet Goldhor. *The Dance of Intimacy.* New York: Harper & Row, 1989.

Minkler, Meredith, and Kathleen M. Roe. *Grandmothers as Caregivers: Raising Children of the Crack Cocaine Epidemic.* Newbury Park, CA: Sage Publications, 1993.

Pasztor, Eileen Mayers, Donna D. Petras, & Cassaundra Rainey (2012). *Collaborating with Kinship Caregivers: A Research to Practice, Competency-Based Training Program for Child Welfare Workers and Their Supervisors*. Washington, DC: Child Welfare League of America. 2012.

Poe, Lenora Madison. *Black Grandparents as Parents*. Berkeley, CA: Lenora Madison Poe, 1992.

U.S. House of Representatives, Committee on Ways and Means. *2008 Green Book: Overview of Entitlement Programs*. Washington, DC: U.S. Government Printing Office, 2008.

———. *2011 Green Book*. Washington, DC: U.S. Government Printing Office, 2011.

U.S. Senate, Committee on Labor and Human Resources, Subcommittee on Children, Family, Drugs, and Alcoholism. *Falling through the Crack: The Impact of Drug-Exposed Children on the Child Welfare System* (hearing, March 8, 1990). Washington, DC: U.S. Government Printing Office, 1990.

BROCHURES/PAMPHLETS/PAPERS

Center for Law and Social Policy and Children's Defense Fund, together with 16 collaborating national organizations. *New Help for Children Raised by Grandparents and Other Relatives: Questions and Answers about the Fostering Connections to Success and Increasing Adoptions Act of 2008,* January 2009. Available at Children's Defense Fund website, *www.childrensdefense. org*, under Research Library.

Centers for Disease Control and Prevention. *Attention Deficit/Hyperactivity Disorder (ADHD): Data & Statistics.* Washington, DC: Centers for Disease Control and Prevention, 2010. Available at *www.cdc.gov/ncbddd/adhd/data.html.*

Chicago Legal Advocacy for Incarcerated Mothers. *When a Parent Is Arrested: Caring for the Children.* Chicago, IL: Chicago Legal Advocacy for Incarcerated Mothers, 2009.

Child Welfare Information Gateway. *Adoption Assistance for Children Adopted from Foster Care.* Washington, DC: U.S. Department of Health and Human Services, Children's Bureau, 2011.

———. *Consent to Adoption.* Washington, DC: U.S. Department of Health and Human Services, Children's Bureau, 2010.

Guttmacher Institute. *Facts on American Teens' Sexual and Reproductive Health.* Accessed February 2012 from *www.guttmacher.org/pubs/FB-ATSRH.html.*

———. *Substance Abuse During Pregnancy, State Policies in Brief, 2012.* Accessed May 1, 2012, from *www.guttmacher.org/statecenter/spibs/spib_SADP.pdf.*

Judicial Council of California. *Guardianship Pamphlet, JV-350* (July 1, 1989).

Legal Aid Foundation of Los Angeles Government Benefits Unit. *The Foster Care Manual.* Los Angeles, CA: Legal Aid Foundation of Los Angeles, 1993.

National Information Center for Children and Youth with Disabilities. *Learning Disabilities* (Fact Sheet Number 7). Washington, DC: National Information Center for Children and Youth with Disabilities, 2011.

Perkins, Jane. *Advocate's Medicaid EPSDT Reference Manual.* Chapel Hill, NC: National Health Law Program, 1993.

The Sentencing Project. *Incarcerated Parents and Their Children: Trends 1991-2007.* Washington, DC: Sentencing Project, February 2009.

Social Security Administration. *Benefits for Children with Disabilities* (SSA Pub. No. 05-10026) (brochure). Baltimore, MD: Social Security Administration, June 2011.

———. *Supplemental Security Income (SSI)* (SSA Pub. No. 05-11000) (brochure). Baltimore, MD: Social Security Administration, May 2011.

———. *Survivors Benefits* (SSA Pub. No. 05-10084) (brochure). Baltimore, MD: Social Security Administration, April 2011.

Superintendent of Documents, U.S. Government Printing Office. "The Abuse of Prescription and Over-the-Counter Drugs." Washington, DC: U.S. Government Printing Office. Accessed October 24, 2012. Available at *http://theanti-drug.com/pdfs/resources/teen-rx/Prescription_Abuse_brochure.pdf.*

U.S. Department of Health and Human Services. *Mental Health: A Report of the Surgeon General.* Rockville, MD: U.S. Department of Health and Human Services, Substance Abuse and Mental Health Services Administration, Center for Mental Health Services, National Institutes of Health, National Institute of Mental Health, 1999. Available at *http://137.187.25.243/library/mentalhealth/chapter3/sec4.html.*

U.S. House of Representatives Committee on Ways and Means. *2008 Green Book.* Washington, DC: U.S. Government Printing Office. Accessed October 19, 2012. Available at *http://waysandmeans.house.gov/media/pdf/111/s111cw.pdf.*

———. *2011 Green Book.* Washington, DC: U.S. Government Printing Office. Accessed October 19, 2012. Available at *http://greenbook.waysandmeans.house.gov.*

MAGAZINES/NEWSPAPERS/JOURNALS

Accinelli, Laura. "Starting Over," *Daily Breeze* (Torrance, California), September 11, 1988.

Angel, Sherry. "Starting Over: Grandparents Who Step In and Raise Their Grandchildren," *Los Angeles Times/Orange County,* April 15, 1991.

Beal, Eileen. "Grandparents Raising Grandchildren," *Cleveland Jewish News,* November 23, 1990.

Creighton, Linda L. "Silent Saviors," *U.S. News & World Report,* December 16, 1991.

Dobbin, Muriel. "Grandmothers Fill In for Drug-Abusing Parents," *Senior Highlights,* March 1990.

Dunn, Ethel. "Those Wonderful Abuelas," *Intergenerational Hookup,* Winter/Spring 1993.

Durkin, Miriam. "When Grandparents Start Over," *Charlotte Observer,* November 3, 1991.

"Eight Famous Persons with Learning Disabilities," *Their World,* January 1981.

"Family 'Kin Care' Trend Increasing," *NASW News,* May 1992.

Girion, Lisa, Scott Glover, and Doug Smith. "Drug Deaths Now Outnumber Traffic Fatalities in U.S., Data Show," *Los Angeles Times,* September 17, 2011. Available at *http://articles.latimes.com/2011/sep/17/local/la-me-drugs-epidemic-20110918.*

Greene, Karen. "The Great American Grandparent: Reinventing Families," *Children's Advocate,* March/April 1992.

Haas, Jane Glenn. "It Can Be Grand to Be Raised by Grandparents," *The Orange County Register,* March 25, 1992. Available in the archives at *www.ocregister.com/articles/archives-218862-county-orange.html.*

Harris, Warren. "Raising a Second Family," *Las Vegas Sun,* June 19, 1989.

Harris-Dawson, Marqueece. "For Grandparents Day, let's support the care they give," *The Sacramento Bee,* September 9, 2011.

Heimpel, Daniel. "Children of the System," *The Daily Beast/Newsweek,* March 8, 2009.

Hornbaker, Alice. "Parents Second Time Around," *Cincinnati Enquirer,* September 10, 1991.

Housen, Patty. "Retiring to the Nursery: Grandparents Raising Kids' Kids," *Senior Beacon: In Focus for People over 50,* May 1990.

Johnson, Trish. "'Older' Parents Need Support," *Katy Times,* February 25, 1990.

"Legal Rights Because of Learning Disabilities," *L/D Law,* 1990.

Lin, Judy. "Recruit in War on Drugs Has Own Battle Scars," *Los Angeles Times,* March 22, 1999.

Link, Tony. "When Kids Come to Grandma's House to Stay," *Daily News* (Los Angeles, California), December 19, 1989.

Malcolm, Andrew H. "Helping Grandparents Who Are Parents Again," *The New York Times,* November 19, 1991. Available at *www.nytimes.com/1991/11/19/nyregion/our-towns-helping-grandparents-who-are-parents-again.html.*

Martin, Richard. "Prescription Drug Epidemic Spreads to Babies," *St. Petersburg*

Times (now *Tampa Bay Times*), July 18, 2010. Available at *www.tampabay.com/news/health/article1109348.ece.*

McDaniel, JoBeth. "The Second Shift," *Life,* June 1, 1992.

Miller, Jeffrey. "Woman Fights Social Service Agencies," *Los Angeles Times,* January 3, 1988.

Moyer, Christine S. "ADHD Rises 32% among Children and Teens," *American Medical News,* September 2, 2011. Available at *www.ama-assn.org/amed-news/2011/08/29/hlsb0902.htm.*

Palmer, Ellen. "Grandparents Raising Grandchildren—The Golden Years: Cancelled," *Valley Magazine* (Orange County Beach Cities, California), December 1990.

Park, Alice. "Teens and Drugs: Rite of Passage or Recipe for Addiction?" *Time,* June 29, 2011.

Pollack, Susan R. "The Grandparent Trap," *The Detroit News,* July 17, 1991.

Smolowe, Jill. "To Grandma's House We Go," *Time,* November 5, 1990.

"Study: 22 Million Americans Use Illegal Drugs," *CNN Health,* September 8, 2011. Available at *http://thechart.blogs.cnn.com/2011/09/08/study-22-million-americans-use-illegal-drugs-3.*

Swartz, Susan. "When Grandparents Are Parents Again," *Press Democrat* (Santa Rosa, California), July 14, 1991.

Toufexis, Anastasia. "Innocent Victims," *Time,* May 13, 1991.

Watson, Ingrid. "Rocking the Cradle," *Fort Worth Star-Telegram,* November 13, 1988.

Welner, Melissa Balmain. "A Testament to Survival," *Orange County Register,* June 14, 1992.

Wild, Madeleine. "Grandmas Forced to Become Moms," *Woman's World,* July 16, 1991.

Wilson, Mary Lou. "Recycled Parents," *The Reporter* (Vacaville, California), March 19, 1990.

Worthington, Robin. "The Second Time Around," *San Jose Mercury News,* March 22, 1992.

Yorkey, Mike. "Picking Up the Pieces," *Focus on the Family,* September 1993.

Zupan, Fran H. "Love Is Grand," *State Newspaper* (Columbia, South Carolina), April 9, 1992.

PRESS RELEASES

Centers for Disease Control and Prevention. "Prescription Painkiller Overdoses at Epidemic Levels. Kill More Americans Than Heroin and Cocaine Combined." Centers for Disease Control and Prevention, Atlanta, GA, November 1, 2011.

Glaze, Lauren E., and Laura M. Maruschak. "Parents in Prison and Their Minor Children." U.S. Department of Justice, Bureau of Justice Statistics, Special Report, 2008.

Johns Hopkins Medical Children's Center. "Children Who Lose a Parent to Suicide More Likely to Die the Same Way." Baltimore, MD: Johns Hopkins Medical Children's Center, April 21, 2010.

Leadership Council on Child Abuse and Interpersonal Violence. "How Many Children Are Court-Ordered into Unsupervised Contact with an Abusive Parent after Divorce?" Baltimore, MD: Leadership Council on Child Abuse and Interpersonal Violence, September 22, 2008.

Office of the Press Secretary. "President Names Members to the Commission on Drug-Free Communities." Washington, DC: The White House, Office of the Press Secretary, October 30, 1998.

MISCELLANEA

89.3KPCC (Southern California Public Radio). "The Power of 3 Extra Years: AB12 to the Rescue of California's Foster Youth, October 1, 2010. Available at *www. scpr.org/programs/patt-morrison/2010/10/01/16285/ab12-signed.*

California Welfare and Institutions Code Section 313. Accessed October 25, 2012. Available at *http://law.onecle.com/california/welfare/313.html.*

ChildHelp. *National Child Abuse Statistics,* accessed May 25, 2012. Available at *www.childhelp.org/pages/statistics.*

Code of Federal Regulations. 34 C.F.R. § 300.321.

Donahue. April 11, 1991.

Gateway Recovery Services and the Pathology Department of Borgess Hospital. *Drugs of Abuse Information Sheet.* Available at *www.ncsconline.org/wc/publications/res_judedu_substanceabusematerial19pub.pdf.*

Individuals with Disabilities Education Act. 20 U.S.C. 1400 et seq.

National Center on Substance Abuse and Child Welfare. *Substance-Exposed Infants.* Accessed March 2012. Available at *www.ncsacw.samhsa.gov/ resources/substance-exposed-infants.aspx.*

Rehabilitation Act of 1973. 29 U.S.C. 794 et seq., § 504.

Seniors Speak Out, KPBS TV, San Diego, November 26, 1992.

Social Security Act, Title IV-E, 42 U.S.C. 670 et seq., § 475.

Index

319

About the Authors

Sylvie de Toledo, LCSW, BCD, is Founder and Clinical Director of Grandparents As Parents, Inc., a nonprofit organization based in Los Angeles, California, and is a recognized expert on issues affecting grandparents and other relative caregivers. She has received awards and other honors from organizations including the Alliance for Children's Rights, the Southern California Psychiatric Society, the United States Senate's Special Committee on Aging, and the California Coalition of Relative Caregivers. She lives in Los Angeles with her husband and daughters. Her website is *www.grandparentsasparents.org.*

Deborah Edler Brown is an award-winning journalist and poet based in Los Angeles. She was a long-time reporter for *Time* magazine and has written for numerous other publications, including *Psychiatric Times.*